I0711575

Mindfulness Meditation for Kids

A Complete Guide for Kids, With Daily Exercises to Relieve Stress, Anxiety, Build Responsibility and Promote Peacefulness and Positive Thinking

LILLY ANDERSEN

© Copyright 2020 - All rights reserved.

The content contained within this book may not be reproduced, duplicated or transmitted without direct written permission from the author or the publisher.

Under no circumstances will any blame or legal responsibility be held against the publisher, or author, for any damages, reparation, or monetary loss due to the information contained within this book. Either directly or indirectly.

Legal Notice:

This book is copyright protected. This book is only for personal use. You cannot amend, distribute, sell, use, quote or paraphrase any part, or the content within this book, without the consent of the author or publisher.

Disclaimer Notice:

Please note the information contained within this document is for educational and entertainment purposes only. All effort has been executed to present accurate, up to date, and reliable, complete information. No warranties of any kind are declared or implied. Readers acknowledge that the author is not engaging in the rendering of legal, financial, medical or professional advice. The content within this book has been derived from various sources. Please consult a licensed professional before attempting any techniques outlined in this book.

By reading this document, the reader agrees that under no circumstances is the author responsible for any losses, direct or indirect, which are incurred as a result of the use of information contained within this document, including, but not limited to, — errors, omissions, or inaccuracies.

Tables of Contents

Introduction

Meditation is not only about sitting in silent concentration, although it is central to the practice. It's also about a series of active techniques that enhance the mind-control ability that is used not only during this sitting, but also in the rest of the awake (and perhaps even the dreaming) life. Meditation thus touches on most aspects of human experience, making them potentially richer, deeper, and productive.

In one form or the other, meditation has been practiced by all the great spiritual traditions, and their origins are lost in the fog of time.

Some of the early teachings on the basic technique of meditation (breathing observation) were made by the Buddha around 500 BC. Patanjali, the semi-legendary founder of Yoga philosophy, offers even more details about the Yoga Sutras, which date back to the second century BC. The unbroken tradition of meditation goes from Patanjali to the present day, where more people than ever have meditated.

Meditation is essentially a state of balanced, high-leveled

concentration that is not focused on a thought or idea train, but on a single, well-defined stimulus. Meditation is the opposite of wandering thoughts or even of a directed train of thought. Buddhaghosa, a fifth-century Buddhist monk, spoke of meditation as a training of attention. Other early authors have more generally referred to it as training the mind or as a way to dig and analyse what is going on in the mind. Over the years, other authors have defined meditation in various ways, as a standstill of the mind, a concentration of mental energy, a discovery of the true self, attainment of inner peace, harmonization of body and mind, or simply sitting still and doing nothing. But it is a very special way to sit still and do nothing in which the mind is kept clear and still, alert and watchful and free from losing oneself in thought.

Phrases like training the mind are a surprise to many Westerners. Isn't our formal education system in schools and universities meant for training of the mind? Isn't' the mind being trained by learning the facts, figures, and techniques of the various academic subjects being taught by our teachers and faculty?, Why should we have to deal with something as seemingly esoteric and time-wasting as meditation?.

Unfortunately, the mind is not quite categorically trained by the facts and figures and techniques taught in our school and universities. The knowledge we acquire over these years is of tremendous value to us and in many cases, to our fellow human beings, but it is not spiritual training.

Anyone who is still in doubt can go ahead and do a simple test. Close your eyes and stop thinking……

How did you progress? Very few people can handle a seemingly simple task for half a minute. So, who is responsible for your mind? One thing is for sure, if you cannot stop thinking for 30 seconds, you certainly are not thinking.

We tend to think that "thinking" is a good thing, provided we have some control over the manner in which ideas are created and the direction to which they are going.

Chapter 1.   An Introduction To Mindfulness

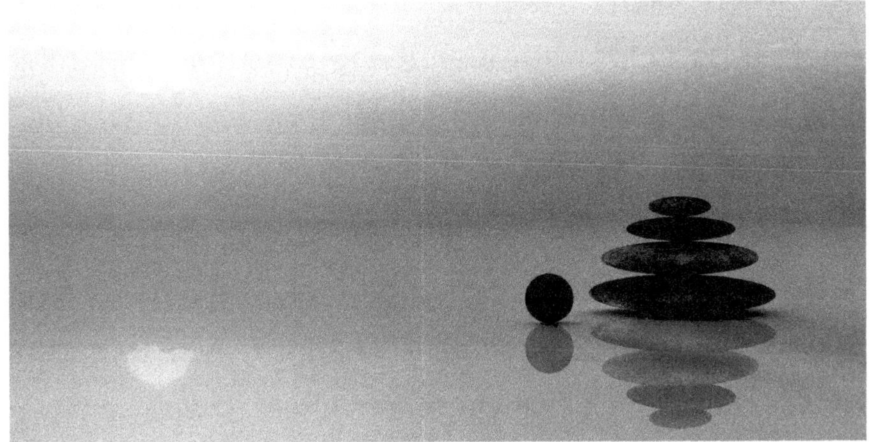

Many people are guilty of doing things quickly, without thought. When you are not focused on the things you are supposed to or whatever is stressing you out, you experience life more fully. Mindfulness is about not worrying about the past or future but being aware of the moment. By living in this way, you can invite calm and rational thought into your life. You learn critical skills that can benefit you through life, and so will your child. Here are some of the benefits.

General Benefits of Mindfulness

#1: Better Decision Making

Mindfulness helps with identifying emotions that might hinder the decision-making process. Have you ever been tired or stressed and made a poor decision? For example, your spouse may have done something to upset you. Instead of confronting them, you make assumptions and lash out. You decide to be passive aggressive, 'forgetting' to pack them lunch or giving them short, snappy answers when they ask you how your day went.

Instead, you could decide to confront them. Tell them what you know and ask them what they have to say about the situation. Think about it critically and decide if they are telling the truth. Then, take deep breaths and decide how to respond. Yelling does not solve anything— you must decide if you are going to forgive them and move forward or respond in another way. For example, if they cheated, you might decide to end the relationship.

#2: Improved Social Interactions

Both children and adults can benefit from improving their social interactions. Mindfulness teaches a deeper connection to emotions. It helps teach empathy. This empathy helps us understand ourselves and not be so critical, but it also helps us understand others. This deeper understanding can give us an idea of why people may react the way they do in certain situations. It teaches us to be kind to the mother with screaming children in the store or the homeless people on the street because we have no idea what life has handed them.

#3: Ability to Deal with Stress

Life rarely goes the way that we intend it to. It is normal for people to experience problems like job loss, the death of a loved one, sickness, break-ups, and other unpleasant situations in their lifetime. However, the people that succeed in life are those that learn to overcome the stressful situations.

For example, imagine that you lost your job. There is the option that some people turn to—drinking away their worries or finding some way to numb what they are feeling. However, this numbness will not help them find a new job. It is an unhealthy reaction to stress. Instead, the energy spent drinking or numbing the stress can be used constructively to create a resume or fill out job applications.

Mindfulness Benefits for Children

In addition to the general benefits of mindfulness, there are specific advantages of teaching your child mindfulness.

#1: Their Minds Are Less Busy

Have you ever reflected on your childhood, wishing you could go back to a time when everything was simpler? As you age, responsibilities grow and there is increased pressure from the world to keep busy. Even high school students have more responsibility than younger children, having to juggle extra-curricular activities, homework, and a social life. Once children grow into adults, their minds become busy places where you cannot enjoy what you are doing sometimes because you are worried about the future.

Children's minds are a little less busy than the average adults. Their parents shoulder a lot of the responsibilities, so they can focus on being a child. Learning mindfulness from a young age is beneficial because children's minds are a less busy place. It can make learning mindfulness a little easier for them.

#2: They Learn to Regulate Their Emotions Better

Most parents will tell you that the terrible twos are a real thing. However, they typically roll over into the terrible threes, fours, and so on. This is a coming of age that exists because toddlers are learning their emotions for the first time. They are starting to find their place in the world and when the world does not fall into place the way that they want it to, it causes them to become sad, angry, and upset.

Teaching children mindfulness also teaches them emotional regulation. As they learn about the different emotions, as well as the thoughts and physical feelings that go along with them, they learn how to better manage these emotions. They also learn techniques for handling stress and other negative emotions, such as the Squish and Release technique that will be covered in the second section of this book.

#3: Increased Ability to Focus

Cognitive focus is something that benefits anybody, but it is especially helpful for children. Kids often have high levels of physical energy than adults. Even though they may not have to juggle as many tasks, their minds often race and become easily distracted. By increasing your child's ability to focus by encouraging mindful practice, you are giving them a better chance at academic success. They will be able to calm themselves better and focus on the task at hand.

#4: Improved Self-Esteem

Kids of any age are at a critical point in their lives that can shape their future. One major struggle that some kids have is with their self-esteem. This can cause them to doubt their abilities, struggle in school, or even become victims of bullying.

The way that mindfulness helps is because it teaches children not to listen to the negative thoughts in their head. Often, there is a voice of self-doubt. When we make a mistake, it might say that we are 'stupid' or 'incapable.' This is far from the truth—everyone makes mistakes. Mindfulness gives children the rational thought to overcome this voice, as well as the voice of bullies and other critics that might hold your child back from being all that they can be.

How to Practice Mindfulness

Plot twist: You actually already know how to be mindful! While you read this sentence, notice your awareness of the following: the meaning of the words, the sounds you hear around you, the thoughts in your head, and the rhythm of your breathing. Congratulations—you just practiced mindfulness! Mindfulness meditation just means doing this deliberately.

To break it down further, mindfulness is the practice of paying attention to what's happening right now in your mind and body in a kind, interested, and nonjudgmental way. It allows you to be aware of what's happening as it happens, rather than getting caught up in stories, judgments, or worries about what did, might, could, or should be happening. Once you have that awareness, you can respond to what's going on in a way that you choose rather than reacting on autopilot. Mindfulness trains you to focus on what you want when you want and to ground your attention in your body and senses, so you don't get carried away with thoughts and emotions (if you don't want to).

It's all about that feeling when you want to give up, because your brain is telling you that you're too ugly, too fat, too dumb, or too skinny; when you can't sleep at night because your mind will not settle down; when you actually did something great but feel like you don't deserve any praise or love; or when you start to freak out because someone didn't message you back. If you've experienced those or similar feelings, you know how your automatic reactions aren't always helpful. Mindfulness lets you train your mind to see what's happening in a way that's appreciative rather than judgmental, and accepting rather than resistant or analytical. That perspective lets you be kinder to yourself as you look in the mirror, get more rest because you can let go of worries more easily, feel the pride of your accomplishments or enjoy the love you deserve, and be more patient with yourself and others when you aren't getting the response you wanted.

At its best, your mind is amazing. It lets you learn, solve problems, play sports, try new things, and more. At its worst, your mind can be like an Internet troll—judgmental, mean, quick to argue, and UNRELENTINGLY LOUD. It can also be like an overzealous therapist, analyzing every little thing you do, obsessing about the past or what's coming next or why things ended up this way. Mindfulness is like a friend, teacher, or parent who tells you that you're doing great, this too shall pass, and you don't have to listen to that shouting jerk or the nattering worrier. Mindfulness trains you to be here now, just as you are, and know that that's okay. As cheesy as it sounds, it's about being a friend to yourself and your experiences rather than needing to change them, get rid of them, or believe the voice that says you're not good enough.

How It Can Help You

This is not about "fixing" yourself or getting rid of who you are. It's about relating to yourself and the world around you in a way that promotes your own happiness and well-being. It doesn't mean that life will suddenly be perfect, but rather that you can be kinder to yourself when everything feels wrong. It's actually really empowering, because you get to be in charge of your mind rather than it being in charge of you.

Sadly, the superpowers of mindfulness are limited. It won't make exams, curfews, demanding bosses, mean people, or unrealistic body standards go away. It can't do much about racism, homophobia, or sexism on a broad scale. But it can help you deal with all of that in a way that makes your life easier, letting you find more compassion for yourself and other people. Instead of hating the exam, calling yourself dumb, or being sure you're going to fail, mindfulness lets you just take the exam. It lets you see what's happening for what it is (nerves, mistakes, pain, discomfort, frustration, distracting thoughts) without adding extra stress. The goal isn't to make those pains or discomforts go away (which is usually out of your control, anyway), but to see that they are actually just uncomfortable feelings that won't last forever. You might still be stressed, but you won't be stressed out.

You can't change a lot of what happens to you. You can't change the past, mistakes you've made, much of what you look like, where you're born, etc. But, if you can see and acknowledge those experiences, then you can decide how you want to relate to them. With practice, you can live your life in a way that lets you accept what you can't change and have the strength and compassion to be the person you want to be.

Neuroscientists are discovering more and more about how our brains can grow and change based on our experiences and habits. Basically, your brain gets good at what it practices. This concept, called neuroplasticity, is what meditation is all about. You probably weren't very good the first time you picked up a violin, hopped on a skateboard, or attempted a three-pointer—but the more you practiced, the better you got. Your brain works the same way. The more you engage in self-criticism, catastrophizing, and judging yourself and others, the better you'll become at those reactions; they'll become more automatic and will be easier to access whether you like them or not. The good news is that every time you pause before reacting, take a breath, are kind to yourself, focus on your good qualities more than the bad, or forgive yourself for making a mistake, the more those habits will become a part of who you are. By reading this book and completing these exercises, you are choosing how you will train your brain and what kind of person you will be.

What to Know before You Start

Reading about mindfulness is like reading about music— you can't get the full experience only through books. To get what mindfulness is all about, you have to try it.

These can be applied to almost every part of your life. They cover everything from using your breathing to focus your attention, to dealing with emotions and thoughts skillfully, to cultivating gratitude and self-compassion. The rest of the book addresses specific scenarios. Each practice includes one of four tips:

•Buddy Up: how to do the practice with a friend, family member, or partner

•Change It Up: ways to vary the practice

•Take It Further: how to dive deeper and explore the practice further

•Am I Doing This Right?: helpful hints and suggestions, or common obstacles

Responding Vs. Reacting And Expectations Vs. Intentions

These meditations build the basic skills for mindfulness. You're training yourself to respond rather than react. Mindfulness teacher Sam Himelstein describes the difference: "Responding is when you think before you act. Reacting is when you act before you think."

When I started meditating, I noticed that I had lots of automatic reactions about meditation itself. It was a combination of "this is amazing, it's going to solve all my problems," "this is a huge waste of time," and "why am I the only one who can't do it?"—none of which was all that helpful for simply being in the present moment.

The ability to respond rather than react can have life-changing, real-world implications. I've worked with teens who use these tools to stay focused while being taunted by competitors at major sporting competitions. Others were able to walk away from a fight rather than get sucked in. One student told me about a time she was able to pause and change her mind before hurting herself. In a society where you're judged and targeted for things you can't control, like your sexuality, the color of your skin, or your body or gender identity, being able to choose how you respond can be the difference between well-being and stress—or even safety and danger.

Having said that, it's important to let go of expectations. Of course, you wouldn't be reading this book if you didn't want to get something from it. But the somewhat annoying and totally paradoxical thing about meditation is that the more expectations you have and the more you try to make something happen, the less likely it is to happen.

It's like when you tell yourself to calm down or someone tells you, "Cheer up, stop being so stressed." Does it work? Almost never. The best way to actually calm down or stop stressing is to respond rather than react, to have intentions rather than expectations. Instead of fighting the stress or expecting to feel something different, you can acknowledge it with kindness. The stress might not go away, but you aren't beating yourself up for something you can't control or getting mad because it doesn't fit with how your brain thinks things should be. The best way to approach meditation is to be with what's happening rather than trying to get somewhere else.

Key Things To Remember

1. You Can't Do It Wrong. The whole point is to notice what's happening as it's happening. Even if the thing you notice is the thought "this is stupid," that still counts.

2. If You Think Of It As Homework, It Feels As Crappy As Homework. Try to think of it as a break or a rest instead. It's a time to chill out rather than another thing to do or get right.

3. The Goal Is Not To Make Everything Happy Or Calm. That means that whatever you feel is okay. Mindfulness isn't about making yourself feel any particular way, and it's not about stopping how you currently are. It's just seeing (and hearing, smelling, tasting, touching, thinking, and feeling) what's happening as it happens.

4. Mindfulness Isn't Asking You To Sit Back And Let The World Walk All Over You. If you want to change something, you still get to change it. Ultimately, you can't change anything without seeing it first. Mindfulness helps you do that.

5. You Definitely Won't Stop Thinking When You Meditate! It's not about making your mind go blank or getting rid of thoughts. It's just noticing what's happening and choosing how much and what kind of attention to give it. Everyone's mind wanders.

6. If You Ever Feel Overwhelmed By What You Experience While Meditating (Or Otherwise), Try To Remember That Even If It Feels Scary Or Really Intense, You Are Okay. You aren't doing it wrong (meditation, or just living in general). If you do get overwhelmed, you might want to open your eyes if they're closed, take a few deep breaths, and use your senses to connect to your environment.

(See here and here for more.)

7. People Call It The Practice Of Mindfulness Or
Meditation For A Reason. Like any skill, it takes practice.
If it feels weird or awkward at first, don't worry. The more
you do it, the more natural it becomes.

Tips for Success

Mindfulness is actually easy. The challenge is
remembering to do it. Use these tips as a way to support
the habit you are trying to build.

Posture Matters. You can meditate in any posture that
feels comfortable. It can help to sit with a straight spine,
a bit more upright and energized than you normally
would. This posture is probably different from how you
usually sit, and it can promote clarity and concentration.
It's better to practice on a straight-backed chair or on a
cushion on the floor rather than on a couch or in bed
(you're less likely to fall asleep). Your eyes can be either
closed or open with a soft gaze such that you aren't really
looking at anything (unless you are doing a practice that
asks you to look around your environment).

Make It A Habit. The best way to make mindfulness,

compassion, and nonjudgment a more permanent part of who you are is to practice regularly. Try to find a regular time when you can practice these meditations (maybe between school and work, between classes, or right before bedtime). At the same time, experiment with practicing informally throughout your day. Anytime you can stop and take a breath is an opportunity to train your brain.

Use A Timer. It's really helpful to choose how long you will meditate for and set a timer (it can even be your phone) for that length of time in advance. Then hide the timer behind you, so you won't be tempted to peek at it. There are lots of free timer apps you can use.

Keep A Journal. A meditation journal is another helpful tool. It can be a fancy notebook or just notes on your phone. Make it as detailed or as brief as you like—for example, "Practiced for five minutes, noticed my mind felt crazy and felt my breath in my nose." The journal helps support the habit and keeps you accountable.

Find Support. Having a friend who knows what you're doing and who can support you is one of the best ways to promote a regular mindfulness practice. You might text each other once a day with a brief reminder like

"Breathe" or "Pause," to share what you noticed when you meditated, or even just send a thumbs-up emoji after you've practiced. Some people really like meditating with others; others prefer to do it alone. Do what works for you.

Also, while this book is a great way to start your mindfulness journey, it's especially helpful to have someone who can guide you in your practice. There are lots of free resources online, including guided meditations. Check out the resources at the end of the book and/or look up teachers or meditation groups in your area. Lots of teachers offer stuff online, too.

Don't Give Up. Some of the meditations will feel like a great fit for you. Others might not. For example, if you have asthma or experience anxiety, paying attention to your breath might be unhelpful. Try to trust yourself, but also don't give up too easily. If it feels challenging, that's totally normal. If it feels overwhelming or painful, trust yourself and choose a different practice or take a break and come back when it feels right.

You Know Yourself Best. Ask yourself what you need to do to make this commitment or to bring yourself back when you lose track. Maybe you need to set reminders on your phone or download an app for this. Maybe you need to write a note for your mirror or schedule it into your calendar. It's like exercise—sometimes you know you should do it even if you don't feel like it. Once you start, chances are you'll keep going.

Chapter 2. How to Teach Mindfulness Meditation to Children

Mind meditation is the practical cleansing of the mind, of witnessing and transcending the mind. Examples of this type of meditation are Buddhist meditation and TM meditation. Focused meditation is the practice of using the mind as a tool for self-healing and internal transplantation. You practice this type of meditation when you are involved in creative visualization, guided images and breathing exercises. Mindfulness-centered meditation is best for children because it allows the child to practice mindfulness through focused and physical relaxation.

As parents, we can start practicing meditation with our children, usually from 4 years old. This constant practice allows your little one to transform meditation into an integral and natural part of his daily life, even during adulthood.

Teaching children is different from teaching adults. Children have less patience, less distance and less ability to sit. On the other hand, they have a more amazing imagination, a feeling of joy and learn, for example.

Why is meditation so important in our lives? Meditation is an important practice to maintain children's balance and ability to cope with stress. As they slowly and slowly find themselves there, children feed themselves with a healthy sense of themselves and, therefore, improve their self-esteem.

Children in each situation will feel a sense of personal power and the ability to defend themselves. You can experience the world apart from a chaotic and winding world of needs and needs. Creating this space for our children to experience relaxation and self-esteem improves the feeling of happiness and the inner understanding that they can really do what they have in mind.

As a result, to teach children meditation effectively, keep the following six principles in mind.

Make it Attractive and Fun

The most important thing when teaching children to meditate is to present forms in a more attractive, fun and attractive way. Never let them get bored. I love that it is a fun activity like a game) and children have to try again.

The principle of "making it fun" means that you should choose techniques that are naturally appealing to children, such as working with their senses and imagination. It also means that you have to adjust the meditation guidelines to make them more attractive.

For example, instead of asking children to "watch you breathe," you can ask them to put a small toy in their belly and drag it up and down. Have them try to move the toy as slowly as possible.

You go there, you just give them a deep breath and don't even notice it! Of course, this approach depends on age. Is your "student" a child 6-9), between 14-14) or a teenager 14-17)? The way you teach a 5-year-old is different from the way you portray an 11-year-old. This meditation training for children needs to apply these principles and techniques to the child's age and personality.

Appeal to Their Imagination

It is difficult for most children to understand abstract concepts. Instead, children enjoy activities that allow them to use their imagination and creativity. So, make sure you involve your imagination in action.

One way to do this is to frame meditation as a challenge. You have to communicate with your creativity and imagination, and that depends a lot on the child. For example: physical rest is a strong door to meditation.

If your child loves action movies, he can create a metaphor like this: "Your soul is like a secret stealthy agent that sometimes wants to disappear. Your mission is to protect him, so follow him in a careful and silent manner. However, be so careful because he could take to his heels in blink of an eye.

Create an Atmosphere of "Lovely Meditation"

Another way is to create an atmosphere of "lovely meditation" at home or at school. Children like to move to another world with different experiences and strange objects. You can say something like: a sacred space, a magical space, and when you enter and follow the meditation, all your things disappear and you feel very relaxed and happy.

Keep It Short

Children do not have to wait 20 minutes on the floor. Therefore, keep the exercise short, especially for children under 10 years. You should never get tired of exercise, but leave the feeling that you want to "want more."

A general guideline is to hold meetings until the child's age, plus one. So, if your child is 8 years old, do the session for a maximum of 9 minutes. To make it more fun, you can use a ring timer program.

Lead for Example

Children learn more by following the instructions below. They like to imitate adults and feel old. Therefore, the best way to teach a child to meditate is to meditate! All areas are striking, so be sure to give a solid example of how to integrate meditation into your daily life.

Let your child feel still while meditating. Finally, he will ask you what you did and then it will be time to teach them. Otherwise, he will increase his curiosity by saying something like: "This is a special exercise that only adults can do, but if you have a good week, I can teach you on Saturday."

<u>Do you want your children to meditate? Be an example.</u>

It also means that you have to meditate with them. Do you want them to be regular in their training? You need to regulate yourself and make meditation a family practice.

Be Flexible and Supportive

At the end of the exercise together, ask them how their experience was. This would be a good plan to draw them what their meditation session is, the experience they have experienced or the "before and after" drawing. This encourages children to express themselves.

Then, confirm what they share. Accept what the child says, even if it is exaggerated, because we leave room for imagination.

Start with Five Minutes of Relaxation at Bedtime

With five minutes to rest at bedtime is easy. The stories presented in the following chapters will help you get started. Create a short break in bed using your imagination and genius to ask your child to imagine a sun just above their head, eliminating stress or worry. This will make your body very calm and relaxed.

Continue with the details of the relaxation waves above and above the body to touch and relax any muscle and body. Children find this very relaxing.

Bring an animal friend to your stage or a lovely cloud where your child can enter. Help your child relieve stress one by one by pressing stress on a nearby balloon and observing the stress and worry of POPs. There are no infinite possibilities for your stories. Your own living imagination makes these possibilities unlimited.

This focused approach helps children in a variety of ways. Children can concentrate better, feel more balanced in their daily lives, are calmer and more comfortable. If we do not teach our children meditation and tranquility, they become a collection of nervous and unhappy energy. Children desperately need a way out of their stress. 69% of children under 10 have trouble sleeping and 76% of school-age children are worried. As responsible parents, we can provide such tools to our children to help them fully realize their life potential.

Tips for Teaching Your Child Mindfulness: Before You Get Started

- 1: Try Mindfulness Yourself

We are our children's role models. If you are constantly yelling when you are upset or you shut down when emotions become overwhelming, your child will see that and mindfulness will be more difficult for them. You will also have a harder time encouraging them to practice mindfulness since it can be hard to do at first and you are not practicing with them.

To practice mindfulness on your own, start by scheduling 5-10 minutes for meditation each day. Find a quiet place where you can close your eyes and relax. Focus on your breathing, inhaling for a count of five and then exhaling for a count of five. Pay attention to how the breath makes your stomach inflate and deflate. If you find yourself distracted, release the thought without judgment and return your focus to your breathing. As time goes on, you will be able to focus for longer periods without your mind wandering. You can even extend the time beyond 10 minutes once you are comfortable.

- 2: Be Mindful During Daily Activities

Over the course of a lifetime, the activities that you do on a day-to-day basis become second nature. For most people, this means that they start to carry out their daily responsibilities in a robotic-like fashion, sometimes letting their mind wander without giving what they are doing a second thought. Have you ever pulled into the driveway of your house and realized you don't remember coming down the last few streets? This is from driving the same way over and over again. The mind goes on autopilot—this is the reason that many accidents happen within three miles of someone's home.

Being mindful during the day simply means being present. It means that instead of letting your mind go on autopilot while driving to work or doing the dishes, you take the time to realize all that is around you. You notice the flower bushes by the park and hear the sounds of the dogs playing there, instead of tuning them out. You feel the way your muscles move while doing the dishes, paying attention to how the way you move your hand removes dirty spots from the dishes.

- 3: Be Sure Your Expectations are Realistic

People who are familiar with mindfulness often associate it with feelings of calmness and relaxation. The idea of a quiet home is enough for any parent to consider practicing mindfulness with their children. You should keep in mind, however, that teaching your child mindfulness does not mean they will be quiet all the time. While you might notice a difference in the number of tantrums and there will be periods of peace, keeping your child quiet should not be the ultimate goal of mindfulness. The goal is to teach your child the skills that will help them become more aware of their experience, both internally and externally. It will help them learn that their thoughts are only thoughts—not something that they must listen to or judge. Though mindfulness can help, your child is likely to still exhibit what could be considered normal kid behavior—tantrums, whining, arguing, and loudness—from time to time.

Overcoming Common Obstacles to Mindfulness

- 1: Your Child Does Not Understand Mindfulness

Not only is mindfulness a big word, it can be a big concept to explain to a child. You cannot explain mindfulness to your child in the way that it has been described in these first couple chapters. Explaining it in a way that makes it seem complex will make your child feel as if they are unable to understand the idea. Without understanding it, they will not be able to find the motivation to practice it.

Keep things simple by explaining mindfulness as awareness. You are teaching your child to be aware. Awareness is feeling things and understanding thoughts as they come, in the present moment. It is knowing what is happening inside of our bodies and minds right now.

- 2: Your Child is Not Interested

Mindfulness is not something that you can just do. Even though mindful practice is meant to induce a state of relaxation, it can be difficult to get your child to be mindful when they are in the middle of a temper tantrum.

It can also be hard to get them interested if they have had a long day at school or have been cooped up because they will have an excess of energy that will make it hard for them to become aware of their present moment.

If your child is not interested in mindfulness or seems to wound up, do not force it on them. It is important that mindful practice is related to positive emotions if you want your child to be motivated enough to do it. If they seem to be too energized, try practicing mindfulness after playing or other physical activity. If you do become frustrated, remember to keep your expectations in check. You should be practicing mindfulness for the benefits—not to achieve a specific outcome.

- 3: You Are in the Habit of Tuning Them Out

Parents lead busy lives, but that does not excuse us from interacting with our child. When your child is talking about something that excites them, give them your full attention. Avoid checking the ping on your phone. If you do need to take a phone call, excuse yourself and then find them when you are done. Encourage them to share with you.

This does not mean that you should allow your child to be rude. There are appropriate and inappropriate times to talk. Teach them the habit of saying 'excuse me' to interrupt other people's conversations. It is okay to ask them to wait before you attend to them, but do not neglect to pay attention to them.

If interruptions are a problem, then get in the habit of setting aside time for your little one to share about their day with you. It does take more than five to ten minutes. Try to avoid doing this right after school, unless they initiate it. Some kids are excited to share after school, while others prefer to keep to themselves for a while and relax before sharing.

Chapter 3. Techniques And Trips To Relieve Stress And Promote Peacefulness

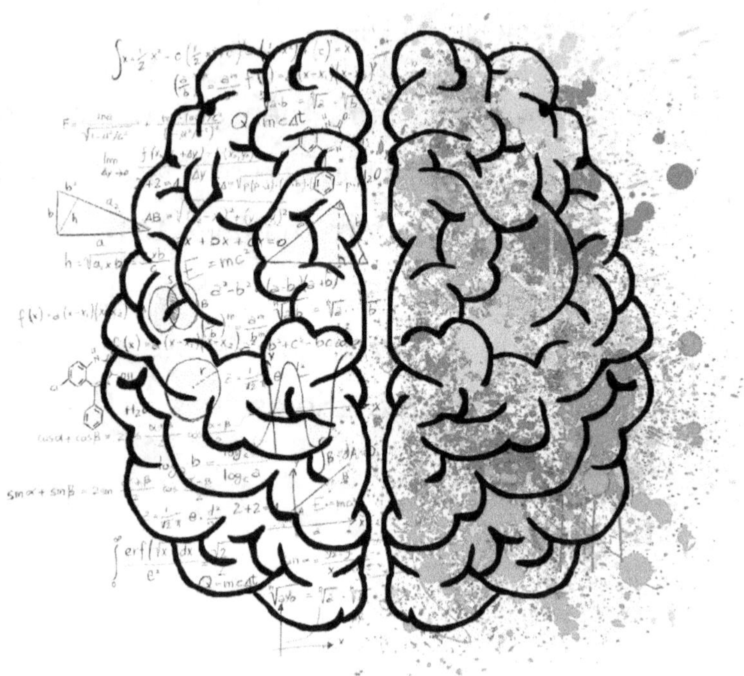

The first 3 steps of practicing mindfulness meditation are the same as the ones you practiced in concentration meditation to relieve stress and promote peacefulness. These steps are: choose a calm place, relax and set a timer. You also need to be seated in a position that respects your spine. Thus, if you are on a hard chair, sit up straight so that energy can pass down to your energy points. Place your feet flat on the floor. If you want to feel even more grounded, kick your shoes off and feel your naked feet on the floor.

Since I have mentioned each step in detail previously, I am not repeating them again. Here are the additional steps you need to perform to become mindful at all times.

It is also a good idea to write down what you want to gain from your meditation and writing in your journal before you start meditation will help to guide your meditation and help you to solve problems that relate to your self-esteem or the problems that present themselves in your life.

• Settle Your Mind: Once you sit comfortably feeling relaxed, detach your mind from all the thoughts of the things going on in your life. It might take a while for you to completely forget everything going around especially if you had a stressful day.

If such is the case, you will notice that your mind is dancing from one thought to another. Don't force it to calm down; just let the thoughts be. Let it dance for a while and once it settles down, bring your focus to meditation, which at the start may feel a strange concept to you but it's okay if you feel this way. Again, if you filled out your thoughts in your meditation book, don't let them go further by continuing to think of them. Just acknowledge that they are there but give them no more credence than that. They are just thoughts.

• Use Your Breath to Become Focused: Once your mind is settled down and your focus is totally on meditation, bring your awareness to your breath as you take it.

Focus on the inhalations and exhalations of each breath. Feel how the air enters your nostrils and then flows through your windpipe into your lungs and then comes back from your lungs to your windpipe then nose and then gets out of your body. Remember the counting that you did when you did the breathing exercises in this book? These will help you because you need to develop a deep breathing rhythm that is steady and if you need to use counting at the beginning, of course, you can do this until you feel comfortable that the amount of breath is just right.

Your mind may come up with a thought to distract you.

If that happens, ignore it and bring back your focus to your breath. Keep in mind that focusing on the actions you are doing right now is itself a practice to become mindful.

Whenever a thought pops up in your mind, instead of fighting with it, just let it flow. Bring in this alternate thought, "Oh! I need to focus on my breath" and then replace it with the action of focusing on your breath. The thing that you need to learn is to acknowledge a thought rather than pretending it isn't there, and simply tell it to go away because you are busy at this time. When you do that, don't attach any emotions to the thought and view it just like it's a scene that is passing you while you are sitting on a train. Judgment is human failure and when you are able to let go of this in your life, you will find that it's much easier to meditate.

• Explore One Thought At A Time: Once you feel more focused and calm, let yourself a little loose and don't shun away any thought that enters your mind. Now your job is to explore them and know yourself better. If you feel any sensation, emotion or feeling, hold on to it and try to understand it better. Ask yourself questions like 'Why do I feel that way?', 'What exactly happened that made me feel this way?' and similar questions. By asking such questions, you try to identify the reason behind that emotion and thought. Make sure not to label any emotion or thought as good or bad, negative or positive; accept it wholeheartedly. Be very patient with it and use it to know yourself better. After doing it for a few minutes, you'll find something new about yourself and the way you think. For instance, you may discover that you feel you're a failure because you don't work hard and this makes you realize the importance of working hard on your goal. This makes you realize your problem and gives you a fix for it too. When your mind is quiet and thoughts arrive, you can explore them and do this very logically instead of involving your emotions and judgment which is when thoughts go haywire.

Repeat this exercise of mindfulness meditation twice a day for 5-10 minutes per session at the start and increase the timing of each session as you progress. Explore new thoughts daily and understand them better to get a true insight into your mind.

As you do that, try to bring mindfulness meditation into each and every aspect of your life as well. What does that mean? Why am I feeling this way? You are perfectly entitled to acknowledge thoughts but not to let them take over your mind to the extent that they impose emotions upon you. When you find that you have had enough of thoughts, go back to being in the moment, in the breath and concentrate on the breath instead of thinking, shunning the thoughts that you really do not wish to deal with at this time or which you know will make you emotional. You are in control of this moment. You can go back to concentrating on the breath at any time. Just think to yourself that this kind of meditation helps to make you aware of your thoughts and the reasons that they occur. However, try to carry on this line of thinking even after you have meditated, because it helps you to accept thoughts, to process them without emotions and to move on to the next thought in your everyday life.

You will see from the next section that you can bring mindfulness meditation into everyday actions and this helps you as a continuance of your mindfulness meditation sessions to accept life as it is, rather than wishing it was different. We cannot change who we are. All that we can change is our approach to life and mindfulness brings you back into the moment, so you don't miss anything along the way.

Bringing Mindfulness Meditation into Every Aspect of Your

Life

This means that you have to be fully involved in everything you do without thinking of anything else or jumping to another task. If you are reading a book, focus on it completely and don't let your mind wander off in thought to something else. Tell yourself 'I have to focus on the book right now' and try to enjoy each word of it. The more you focus on it, the more you become involved in it. This helps you stay in the present and live each moment of it fully.

Similarly, if you are doing laundry, be fully involved in it, so you do or think of nothing else but the act you're involved in right now. It will take you a little time to be mindful of each moment all the time, but practice will help you get there for sure; and when that happens, you'll unlock a beautiful, happy life that will keep you stress-free at all times.

We were never intended to multi task. It really goes against the natural workings of the brain and when you learn to concentrate totally on everything that you do, it takes a whole load of strain off the mind. You also get more done and can work out your goals and really make an effort to reach them, one step at a time. You can make all kinds of tasks meaningful by paying attention to what it is you are doing. I remember one day cleaning the tiles in the shower and thinking how much they sparkle and shine when in the past I would never really have noticed the fruits of my own labor. It was a moment that I enjoyed as I could see my smiling face in the reflection and had used mindfulness to get me through everything that I had to do before folks dropped in to stay at my house.

While you work on this, do introduce body scan meditation into your routine too. It is an excellent technique to get rid of the stress stuck in your body and become fully relaxed.

Chapter 4.   Daily Exercises

You get a million messages about the person you should be: what you're supposed to look like (big lips, flat abs, perfect eyebrows, and more); how you're supposed to act (tough, smart, funny, not too loud or quiet); and how you're supposed to express your sexual or gender identity. And somehow, amid all of that, you're also supposed to "be yourself." These practices are all about taking care of yourself just as you are. Then you can be in the best frame of mind to decide who you want to be.

Silencing Self-Criticism

Very few of us would talk to others the way we talk to ourselves. We'd never be so harsh or mean. Would you ever call your best friend the names you call yourself? Yet it seems to come naturally to be super self-critical.

Mindfulness helps you see that not only are those thoughts not true, they only have as much power as you give them. This practice lets you see your automatic thoughts without needing to believe them, and then choose a different response.

1. Take a moment to pause and notice what's going on right now. Use your senses to bring yourself into the present moment.

2. Notice any sensations in your body right now, particularly your feet on the floor. Remind yourself that it's okay to feel however you feel. Then keep coming back to the feeling of your breath and your feet. (You might also try the postures in the Self-Soothing Practices.)

3. Instead of focusing on the content of the thought, keep returning to how this moment feels in your body.

4. When you're ready, consider if there are any other ways of seeing this situation. Look for counterevidence. How would your best friend interpret this? How would you talk to your closest friend or family member if they were going through this?

5. Next, try to find a more balanced thought. Your automatic reaction might be, "I'm a loser. I always fail." A balanced response might be, "I made a mistake" or recognizing that you thought you'd fail last time but didn't.

6. The critical thought might not go away, but you don't need to fuel it. Remind yourself that the judgments in your head aren't true, no matter how convincing they are.

7. Keep your attention on your breathing and your body. You might choose to focus on something you're grateful for or even the tiniest thing that went well this week.

TAKE IT FURTHER

Almost everyone has this bully (or monster, demon, or troll) in their brain. However you picture it, it's very convincing, very persuasive, and quite charming. It tells you that it knows how to make you feel or be better, if only you'd listen to it. And it thrives on attention. The more you listen to it, the louder it gets. But here's the truth: It's wrong. It's totally wrong. You don't get better by making yourself feel worse. And while you might never be able to make it go away completely, if you know it's there, if you expect it, then it can't surprise you and knock you off balance as much. Use this practice to really see it. Even give it a name or decide what it looks like. Then the next time it shows up, it's not some immovable force. Instead, it's more like that smelly uncle at Thanksgiving. It's inevitably unpleasant, but you don't need to let it get to you.

Mindful Eating and Moving Mindfully

Have you ever eaten lunch and then forgotten that you did it? Ever walked home from school and didn't remember the walk at all? Or finished a bag of chips without even realizing you were eating? Most of us have had the experience of eating mindlessly or even going to the wrong place because we were distracted by something else. Mindfulness helps us be more present because we are attentive to what's happening as it's happening.

1.Whatever you are doing, take a moment to pause and set the intention to do it mindfully—just that one thing, right now.

2.Take a few deep breaths and notice how your body feels in this moment.

3.Then explore the task at hand with all of your senses.

4.If you're eating, notice what the food looks like, how the light hits it, how it smells, how it feels in your mouth as you chew and swallow. Really take your time with it. Put your fork down between bites. Notice any habits you might have, such as reaching for the next piece before finishing the first one. What is it like to just eat, rather than eating while looking at your phone or even listening to music?

5.If you're walking, notice how your feet feel touching the ground. Hear any sounds that are around or within you. Try to place all of your attention on the feeling of walking. Notice how your muscles and joints propel you forward. It's actually amazing how much goes into keeping you upright and moving.

6.You can try this with any activity. Just use your senses to feel what's happening as it's happening. Whatever you are doing, try to do only that one thing.

7.When your mind wanders, bring your attention back to your senses in this moment.

AM I DOING THIS RIGHT?

This might feel weird at first. Who really pays attention to what walking or eating feels like? But the more you do it, the more you'll likely appreciate those chances to stop and just be. You don't even have to do it for the entire walk or meal. Try it with just a few bites or steps. See what happens when you commit to doing just one thing at a time.

Waking Up Mindfully

Ever wake up and immediately feel like it's going to be a terrible day? Or you grab your phone before you're even fully awake? Those first few moments can help you set the tone for the rest of the day. This practice asks you to take just two minutes before picking up your phone or planning your day to be in your body and orient to your environment, so you can make a choice about how you're going to relate to yourself today.

1.You've just woken up. Notice how your body feels. Enjoy the feeling of not needing to do anything before your day starts. You might also check out the light in the room or the sounds you hear.

2.Take a few deep breaths. You can place your hands on your abdomen to feel your body breathing even more fully. Notice what it feels like to breathe.

3.Let your breathing be natural. Notice any stories or thoughts going through your mind. Send yourself kind thoughts (here) or set an intention for how you are going to be today. You might choose to be kind or compassionate or make someone else feel good. This isn't about ignoring anything negative; it's about choosing what you want to focus on.

4.Take a few more moments to connect to your senses. Notice anything you can hear, smell, see, taste, or touch.

5.When you're ready or it's time to get up, renew your intention for how you want to be today. See if there's even one small thing you can look forward to or appreciate in this moment. Rest your attention on that kindness as you get up and go about your morning.

TAKE IT FURTHER

Each moment is an opportunity to start again. If you wake up feeling grouchy, let yourself feel that, name it, and notice that it moves and changes. Then come back to your body and to deciding how you want to be in this moment. You get to be in charge here.

It's important to know that this isn't about being super-optimistic or ignoring any problems you have. Rather, you're seeing that you get to decide, in every moment, how you are with whatever's happening. Consider how you really want to feel when you get back in bed at the end of the day.

Loving Your Body

Most of us have body-image issues, because we have this

idea that our bodies don't look like they should. We believe we look wrong: wrong skin, height, legs, hair, everything. The amazing thing is that it doesn't matter what hair, skin, or height we have—someone will always say it should be different. It's like it is in elementary school, when no matter what your name is, someone will find a way to make fun of it. You can always choose to find something that isn't good enough.

Loving your body isn't about having the perfect arms, abs, or butt. And it doesn't mean you can't work out or eat healthy. It's about seeing that being kind to yourself makes you feel a lot better than treating yourself like crap and that you can choose which messages you take to heart.

1.Take a few deep breaths. Notice how you feel.

2.Let your breath be natural and turn your attention to what your body feels like.

3.Take some time to feel yourself breathing and try to marvel at the ability of your body to breathe and keep you alive.

4.Notice that your senses are working all the time, giving you information and connecting you to the world. You don't even have to tell them to do anything; they just do it.

5.If you feel down or critical, take some time to notice how that feels inside. Let yourself feel that discomfort as sensations in your body rather than focusing on the thoughts or judgments themselves.

6.Try to avoid making major decisions right now. If your mind is saying, "I hate my body" or "I have the ugliest nose ever," try to notice that, right now, your mind is upset. Right now, you feel angry or sad. Right now, frustration feels this way. And it won't last forever even if it feels like it.

7.Remind yourself that you can't change your body by hating it. That only makes you feel worse. Remember that no one is perfect and pictures only tell part of a story. Imagine you could inhale peace and strength and exhale negativity and anger.

8.Take a few more deep breaths and notice how you feel now. Remind yourself that you are enough, just as you are. You might even say it in your head or out loud: "I am beautiful. I am enough. I am strong." Even if it feels strange or forced, the more you do this, the more you'll build kindness instead of judgment.

CHANGE IT UP

As you're noticing how you relate to your own body, notice if you're stuck in a pattern of checking out or critiquing other people. Observe how that makes you feel. You might try to send a silent compliment instead of a critique. Those kinder thoughts can actually have a very significant impact on your own mood and your relationship to others.

Making Choices about Technology

Did you know that tech companies deliberately make apps as addictive as possible? They spend billions of dollars researching ways to turn our phone use into a habit, something we can't live without even for five minutes. Some people call it "brain hacking." Phones aren't bad inherently, but they do become a problem when we check them without realizing it.

This meditation isn't about getting rid of the phone or social media. It's about recognizing how technology makes you feel and then deciding to use it only because you choose to, not because someone wants you to be addicted.

1.Pause. Take a few deep breaths. Notice how you feel as you breathe deeply.

2.Let your breathing be normal.

3.Take a moment to check in with how you feel as you go on social media or use your phone. What happens to your body and mind when you see someone else's photo or image of a perfect vacation? What thoughts automatically run through your mind? What happens in your body? Notice your jaw, your stomach, and your throat. What sensations can you feel?

4.As you notice how this feels, you might also ask yourself, "How does this post or picture make me feel?" Let the answer come to you.

5.As you keep looking or keep checking your feed, notice if you're always wanting more, comparing yourself, or perhaps telling yourself, "I'll be happy when I look like that . . ." Explore how these truly make you feel inside.

6.Let yourself be interested in this experience. It's not black and white. Observe all the nuances of what happens. Then you can decide how you want to proceed.

CHANGE IT UP

It seems ironic to suggest using an app to see how much you use other apps, but it can be really informative. Find an app that tracks your phone or social media use, and make the commitment to use it for three days. Notice what happens when you see the results. Did you know you were checking your phone that often? Then, you might try an experiment to you limit your phone use for a few days and see what happens. Notice how it feels. (Let your family and friends know what you're doing in advance, so they don't freak out.)

Taking Care of Yourself

Have you ever noticed that you can't focus when you're hungry? Or that your mood totally changes after you've gone for a walk or had a shower? How it's so much easier to get annoyed on an empty stomach? (That's why someone invented the word "hangry"!) It might seem rudimentary, but taking care of your own basic needs can change your mind-set, feelings, moods, emotions, and even levels of pain for an entire day. Use this practice as a way to check in with your basic needs before making judgments of yourself or your life.

1.If you find yourself starting to lose it, getting frustrated, wanting to run away, or getting really down on yourself, try to pause where you are and take a few deep breaths.

2.Let your breathing be natural and notice what you can feel with your senses. Feel your feet on the floor and the air on your skin. Notice what you hear and any tastes in your mouth.

3.Then check in with yourself. Before you judge yourself or give up, try to explore some of these questions:

Have I eaten enough today?

Have I drunk water in the last hour?

Could I use more sleep?

Have I gotten dressed today?

Have I showered?

Have I gone outside? Could I go for a walk?

Do I need a hug or connection with a friend?

Have I had any physical exercise at all today?

4.Whatever you need, make the decision to take care of yourself. If you can't do it right now, make a plan to do so when you are able. Remind yourself that whatever's going through your mind right now, you don't have to take it personally or give it too much focus. It's not you; it's hunger or fatigue or some other part of your system needing attention.

5.Once you tend to what you needed, notice how you feel. Take the time to really enjoy the shower or the glass of water. Explore how the air outside feels or what happens when you do put your phone down and take a nap.

TAKE IT FURTHER

Write yourself a reminder for what you need when you get down. Do you need to wait a few days after starting something new before you make a judgment of it? Do you need to go for a walk when you feel depressed? You might make a playlist of songs that bring your mood up when you need them. Then, next time you're feeling down, you have your own tailor-made prescription for what to do.

What to Do If You Feel Overwhelmed

There is nothing wrong with you if you feel like you can't meditate, you're losing it, or you can't think straight!

Sometimes your nervous system overreacts or gets triggered, which makes you feel overwhelmed or out of control. Whether this happens while you're meditating or during the rest of your day, you can use these techniques to rebalance yourself. Find one or two that feel right to you.

BREATHE: It's annoying, but there's a reason everyone tells you to breathe when you're anxious. A deep breath is a signal to your nervous system that there aren't any threats around.

LONGER EXHALATION: This is the ultimate body hack. If you can lengthen your exhalation, you cue your nervous system to tell your body to chill out. It calls for the release of hormones that relax the whole system. Try to breathe in for a count of three or four and breathe out for a count of six to eight. Find the rhythm that works for you.

ASK YOURSELF: "What's the kindest thing I can do for myself right now? What do I need right now that will be helpful?" Focus on things that are healthy and nonaddictive, like going for a walk, resting, or exercising, rather than turning to something that might feel good in the short term but is actually harmful in the long term (like using technology or social media or mind-altering substances).

FOCUS ON OTHER PEOPLE: Sometimes the best thing you can do is to consider what kindness you could show for someone else right now. It's amazing how focusing on others' happiness gets us out of our own ruts. It doesn't have to be big. Write a note of kindness—saying you're doing great or you got this—and leave it on someone's locker or car. Give a random person a compliment. Even pick up a few pieces of garbage.

FOCUS ON THE MOST NEUTRAL THING IN YOUR BODY: This is usually your feet on the ground. Really put all of your energy and focus into feeling your feet. Notice how many toes you can feel without wiggling them. You might walk slowly to really emphasize the sensations.

FOCUS ON SOMETHING PLEASANT: Find a spot outside a window or in the sky that looks pleasing. Focus on a flower. Or notice the sound of the wind or the sun on your face. Let yourself really soak in those feelings and linger on what is pleasant to your system. See the Soaking in the Good practice.

ORIENT TO YOUR ENVIRONMENT: That means looking around you, specifically moving your head and neck to see in front, to the sides, and behind you. Notice anything that catches your eye.

If overwhelming feelings arise while meditating and you feel fine to keep going, try to be with the feelings for a bit and then come back out again, like dipping your toe in the water before swimming. Try the Self-Soothing Practices.

TYPES OF TOOLS AND ACTIVITIES FOR SENSITIVE KIDS

Meditation Activities:

Here are several exercises and practices you can teach your ADHD child to help bring the body to relaxation – one of which is breathing. These include traditional meditation and the Chinese martial art of tai chi. Simply put, meditation is training a mind to relax so that it can focus on other things afterward. Many self-help books and business books recommend meditation to reduce stress and to prepare the mind for challenging tasks that might bring stress. The type of meditation you should teach your ADHD child should have its focus on helping your child loosen up, mellow out, and calm down.

Here's how to go about it:

- Move the body into a posture that opens the lungs,

as well as stretch and relax the muscles.

•	Close the eyes and envision certain images in the mind, with the objective of stopping the mind from racing or wandering so utmost concentration can be placed on controlled breathing.

Breathing In and Out Activities

The quickest way to change an AHD patient's mood is to change the breathing. Simply by focusing on your breathing, you can halt a cascade of inner events that cause anxiety and stress, both of which reduce your capacity to pay attention.

How to do it

•	Focus your attention on your breath. Notice if it is quick or slow, shallow or deep.

•	Continue breathing in and count to three.

•	Exhale for a count of three. Continue to practice this conscious breathing for two minutes.

Sensory Activities

Poor working memory and forgetfulness are characteristic of children and teens with ADHD. In addition, if their attention was not engaged throughout the instruction, they may not remember a lot of what the teacher presented. Many people with ADHD also have coexisting learning disabilities in auditory or visual sequentiality is an excellent means of helping memorize and recall information. Teach and encourage children to create first- letter mnemonics (acronyms and acrostics), which are very helpful in remembering steps in a process or procedure, a sequence of any kind, or other information.

Pair unfamiliar new vocabulary with similar-

sounding familiar words

This is called the keyword mnemonic technique, which involves looking for ways items go together (perhaps they sound alike or look alike) to help remember. Gratitude Activities

Sometimes it feels like walking on pins and needles. You think you've got it figured out. No tags or tight clothing. You know the lists of foods that wig them out.

Relish in Their Successes

It doesn't matter how small. This not only shows them that you care, but it's a great way to remind them that they can achieve and improve. It's also a good way to remind yourself of the good they do and the progress they make even if they still have a long way to go.

Chapter 5. Tips and Tricks to Improve the Effectiveness of Meditation

Meditation helps you relieve stress regardless of the technique you use to practice it. However, there are some tips and tricks that you can apply to enhance the results and increase its effectiveness. Follow the tips mentioned below to get enhanced results.

1: Meditate Twice a Day

If you want to see great results in a short period, then you need to make meditation a regular practice. The best time to meditate is at sunrise and sunset or 6am and 6pm. At these times, there are hardly any distractions and interruptions around you, which allows you to meditate easily and effectively.

In addition, you need to at least meditate twice a day. The effects of one small session of less than 30 minutes don't last for more than 12 hours. Therefore, to feel peaceful and relaxed at all times, it is best to meditate at least twice daily. If you meditate for around an hour and have quite a hectic routine, it's alright to meditate once a day too. However, make sure to stick to this practice and make it a routine. You can also use meditation during your working day in the manner I have suggested helping to calm you and to help you to concentrate on things that are important to you. Meditation awakens the mind and that can be very useful to you in your lunch break, but be sure to do it before you eat rather than trying to do so afterwards.

Secondly, always meditate at the exact same time. If you meditate at 5pm on the first two days, ensure to meditate at the exact time daily. This practice cultivates consistency and punctuality making you regular with meditation. What you may not realize is that habits are formed by repetition. This is true of any habit and adding the habit of meditation to another daily habit will help. This form of habit stacking has been proven to be very effective. What this means is listing things that you do every day at set times. For example, you get up at a set time – so you can meditate on it. You get home from work at a set time and probably sit down and have a coffee or a tea. You can choose this moment to meditate. The point is that with repetition each day of the habit of meditation it will become second nature and part of your daily routine.

In fact, with practice, you will easily get into meditation without trying too much since your body will know 'it is time to meditate' when that time comes. You should also turn off all distractions during your meditation time so that you can concentrate on just being instead of worrying about whether the phone will go off or someone will knock at the door. By choosing a meditation time, you also get those who live with you accustomed to respecting this time that you put to one side for meditation.

2: Eat something but don't be too full

Try to meditate on an empty stomach to easily focus on the practice. When you have just had a meal, your stomach is full, which often makes you lethargic. If you meditate at this time, you're likely to lose focus on the practice and drift off to sleep instead. You may also find that your digestive system makes it too difficult to sit still in the same position and concentrate on just being. Your stomach may be making noises and uncomfortable in an upright position.

However, if you feel really hungry at the time of your meditation session, then eat something light such as a fruit or a piece of chocolate so you can stay alert and concentrate on your meditation and don't become distracted during the practice due to an empty stomach.

I always take a glass of water into the room with me as well as this may help to stave off any hunger or stop you from craving food during your practice.

3: Meditate at the Same Place

Try to dedicate one place to your meditation spot and don't do anything else there. By practicing meditation at the same spot every day and not doing anything else on that spot, you will naturally feel like meditating whenever you go to that spot. As a result, it will be a lot easier to build a habit of meditating when you have a dedicated spot that makes it very easy for you to get into meditation. As we have already mentioned, having a space set aside for meditation will make you more serious about the practice because you will have devoted the space to something you are trying to incorporate into your life and it will be wasted if you do not use it for that purpose. You may have to make adjustments if you find that you are getting sidetracked by noise or by too much light. You will find that perfect spot and when you do, will see the sense in having one particular place in which to meditate. It helps to reinforce the habit.

4: Minimize Interruptions

Put on a "do-not-disturb" sign on the door of your room

before you start meditating. Also, switch off your cell phone to remain focused; if you can't do that, just put it on the silent mode so there is nothing that holds you back and you can completely focus on your practice. Minimizing interruptions will increase your concentration in your practice resulting in better performance. Let people know that this is a time when you need to be alone and need silence. Most people who are aware that you are doing this for your health will respect that you need to be alone. You can also put your phone on answering machine and place a sign on the door of your house to not disturb you for the next twenty minutes or so.

5: Write your Thoughts before Practicing Meditation

One thing that you are likely to struggle with as a beginner is experiencing distracting thoughts while meditating. You can escape this problem with a simple solution. Before starting the session, write down all the thoughts that cross your mind. By doing this, you tell yourself that you have this thought on record, which you will deal with later when the time is right.

For instance, if you wrote everything that came to your mind including the thought of ironing your clothes as you won't get the time tomorrow as you have to leave for office early, it will be easy for you to focus. In fact, if this thought disturbs you, you can relax your mind by telling yourself that you have it on your notice and you will do it when the time is right. This comforts you and helps you return your attention to meditation.

Follow this writing of thoughts with an additional note of why you are meditating, to try and reinforce the idea. You can also add thoughts of things that you are grateful for before you meditate as this puts you in a positive state of mind.

Moreover, also create your meditation journal. Write down your feelings in it before and after meditating every day to understand how you felt after each session. A meditation journal also helps you to understand your weaknesses, which you can work for the next time. Do go through this journal once every week to track your performance and feel good about yourself. If you feel you're doing a great job, treat yourself to something nice to encourage yourself to meditate regularly and develop a habit of it.

Many people write an introductory prayer for their meditation which reminds them of the purpose of meditation and betterment of their approach. This is useful if you are finding it hard to find the incentive to concentrate over a period of time and feel that your efforts are not paying off. You may not feel the benefits straight away. It takes time and persistence, but once you make this a habit, it is certain that you will enjoy your meditation sessions and use them as a better way to get to know who you are and what you want out of life.

6: Use Mudras to get Enhanced Results

Mudras are hand or body positions that influence your energy, mood and feelings. Mostly, the fingers and hands are held in some position, but your entire body can be used to form a mudra too. Here we will discuss some hand mudras to relieve stress and become happy, as it is believed your fingers have nerve connections that connect to different parts of your brain to produce different emotions. Here are some amazing mudras to let go of stress and become happy and peaceful.

1. Tse Mudra to relieve stress

Tse Mudra is well known and is considered as one of the best mudras to combat anxiety and depression. According to Chinese tradition, this mudra is practiced to drive away stress, sadness, fear and brings good luck. It is said that this mudra also increases your intuitive ability. Given below are images followed by the instructions on how to practice this mudra in your meditation.

• When you're sitting or lying in your comfortable position for meditation, place your thumbs on your thighs.

• Now put your thumb between your little and ring finger as you can see in the first picture. Do this with both hands.

• Now encircle your thumb with your other four fingers as you can see it in the second picture.

• Hold this position in your hands throughout your meditation session.

When you incorporate this mudra, you will notice that your stress levels drop more than when you meditate without this mudra.

2.Ksepana Mudra

It is also a very helpful mudra to improve the effectiveness of meditation as well as to increase your inner peace and happiness. This mudra is known for its magical powers to release all the negativity that is being ingested within your soul. You can use this mudra in your meditation especially in those cases where you had a very bad day and you are flooding with negative emotions. Given below is an image that shows the Ksepana mudra along with instructions on how to incorporate this mudra into your meditation.

•   When you start your session and get a comfortable posture, clasp both hands: all the fingers crossing each other.

•   Then take out both index fingers and join their tips as you can see in the picture above.

•   Now drop your hands pointing to the ground. Hold this position for at least 2 minutes, or you can hold it to the entire length of the session.

You will notice great effects after your session ends as the negative thoughts that were flowing through your mind before the session will have greatly reduced.

3. Prana Mudra

Practicing Prana mudra is a good way to collect energy from the universe. Therefore, you can use this mudra to get energized, brighten up your mood and reduce your stress levels. Use this mudra on days when you feel drained out and you don't feel like doing anything because of the energy deficiency. See the picture and instructions below to learn how to practice this mudra.

•	When you get settled for meditation in your comfortable position, join your thumb little and ring finger together as you can see in the picture above and extend your index and middle finger outwards as shown in the picture.

•	Then hold your hands either in a horizontal or vertical position.

•	Keep holding the posture for at least 5 minutes or for the entire duration of your meditation session. Once you complete your session, you will notice that you feel energy running through your body that was not there when you started your session.

4. Lotus Mudra

Lotus mudra is a symbol of purity. In Buddhism, lotus position of hands is reserved to represent the opening of the heart. When you face rejection; you close your heart by slouching your shoulders and collapsing your chest. In other words, you make yourself unavailable to others when you're in stress which raises the tension between your peers and others close to you. As a result, you feel more stressed out when others neglect you because of your behavior.

By incorporating lotus mudra in your meditation, you open your heart to others and in return others return the favor and show gratitude to you, which ultimately reduces your stress levels and makes you happier than ever.

Use this mudra in cases where you find yourself in stressful situations because others are being rude to you. Given below are the instructions along with an image on how to perform this mudra.

•	When you start your meditation session, join both hands in a way that your thumb meets your other thumb and your baby finger meets your other baby finger and both palms meet each other at the bottom. It will make a position of a flower in bloom.

•	Hold this position throughout your session. You will feel a considerable change in the behavior of your peers and others close to you. When everybody is showing your gratitude, your mood will automatically lighten up and your stress levels go down.

Practice all the mentioned tips and tricks to enhance the effectiveness of your meditation sessions. Whichever route you take to fight your stress and anxiety, just remember one thing- change occurs with time but staying persistent is the key to accomplish and enjoy those changes and turn those temporary changes into everlasting ones. Therefore, keep fighting your stress through practicing meditation regularly and you will ultimately defeat your stress to live a happy and peaceful life.

Chapter 6. Guided Mindfulness Meditations for Deep Sleep

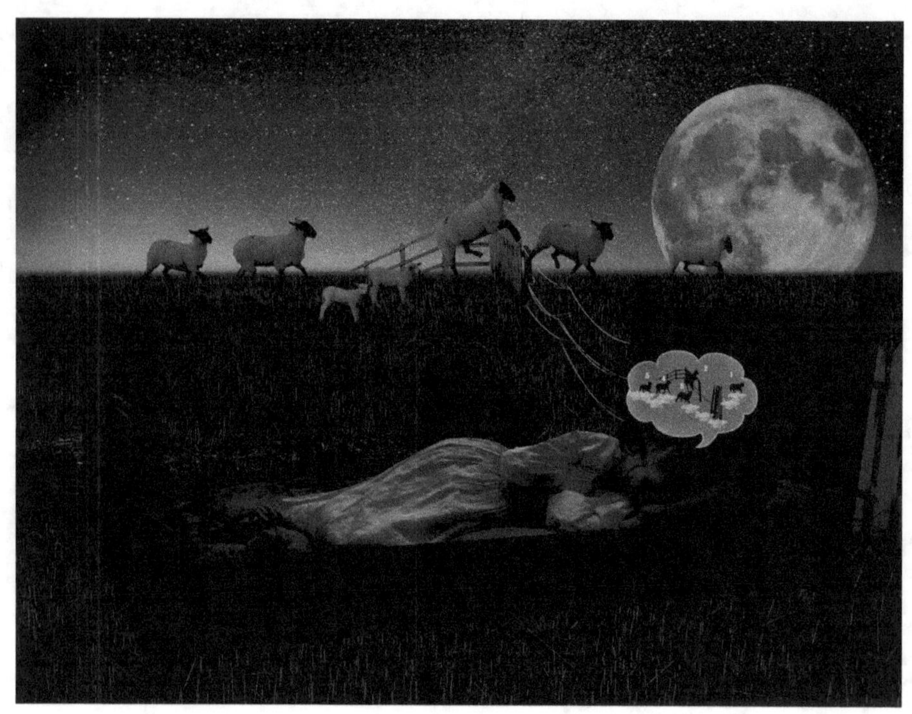

Guide Meditation to Improve Insomnia

Sleep has been a significant issue in the whole world. Many people have insomnia, and this affects their average productive level. Insomnia is a condition feared by many. People who practice mindfulness meditation can fight off this condition. They can fall asleep sooner and stay for long in bed.

Meditation can also reduce pain. It has the power to control any discomfort, be it emotional or psychological. People have perceptions connected to their state of mind. Attitudes like these elevate in the presence of stressful conditions. When you meditate, you will have more activities going on in the part of the brain that controls pain. You will also have less pain sensitivity.

Lastly, meditation is essential in weight loss since it directly involves the mind. The mind will then form perceptions to a particular food as well as start releasing positive thought to healthy food since a healthy mind means a healthy body and soul. Through guided meditation, you can change your eating habits, lifestyle, and even healthy health choices like exercise.

Deciding to stop your bad eating habits is not a onetime thing but can be done gradually by incorporating healthy foods in the diet. The brain triggers the mind to eat, and food cravings also come from the mind. If the mind can accept that there is a need to eat healthily and live positive, so will the brain be triggered towards healthy eating. Weight loss is necessary for healthy living and can keep you away from the many lifestyle diseases, many of which are not curable.

There is a lot of patience involved since it is not the easiest and fastest step towards weight loss but workable none the less. Meditation will help you clear your mind and reduce dependence on food that makes you feel beautiful yet not healthy. This is because the mind is cleared of negative emotions that can be an element of distraction or stress. It is like a painless stress reliever without medication or therapy. It brings weight loss naturally over the long term and creates a very positive and acceptable self-image and self-view.

Guided meditations are not all the same: it depends on the purpose you want to achieve through this practice. Do you just want to relax? Fight insomnia? Become more resilient? Accept a major change? Lose weight?

In most guided meditations, it's essential to try to use as many senses as you can: the smells, the lights, the sounds, the textures. Usually guided meditations have a musical background that invites the mind and body to relax: sounds of nature such as rain, rainforest, sea waves or the sound of a waterfall; or more traditional music like that of the Native American characterized by the sound of flutes, tubes and rattles.

Choose the musical background you prefer, what is important is to create the best condition to relax. To start, you can do a very quick guided meditation for beginners. The basic principle is to pay attention to what you do, always keep it in mind from the beginning to the end of the practice. Close your eyes and start taking three deep breaths, inhaling through your nose and exhaling from your mouth.

When you breathe in you are full of positive energy and when you exhale all kinds of negative energies, such as stress, tension and worries, abandon you. Find your breath and feel your body. Simply observe it (Headspace, n. d.).

Guide Meditation for Depression, Anxiety Relief

Everyone probably experiences stress at some level in their lives. Nearly half of the adult population suffers from its adverse effects. Among these effects include anxiety, depression, arthritis, asthma, high blood pressure, skin conditions, heart problems, and headaches. 75 to 90 percent of doctor visits are because of stress-related issues. When chronic stress is untreated, it can lead to emotional disorder.

Life could really get so stressful, and these days, it's important to find ways to relieve stress without using too much money, or creating more hassle.

One of these ways is hypnotherapy. Research has it that hypnotherapy is one of the best ways of relieving stress, especially for children and teens dealing with anxiety issues. It is said that with the help of hypnosis, feelings of helplessness are lessened and that it's proven to be even greater than that of other traditional relaxation techniques.

It is actually common for kids aged 11 to 15 to develop and experience signs of panic attacks and anxiety. If one wants these experiences to be lessened, he has to learn how to target them right away, then one should at least try going through hypnosis.

A person who has been in a serious automobile accident may have no recollection of it. They may be perfectly fine with no memory loss or impairment. Yet, they are simply unable to recall anything about the accident.

In this case, the conscious mind has taken the memories of a traumatic event, an automobile accident, and archived them in the subconscious mind. By doing this, the mind is protecting the individual from having to relive the traumatic experience over and over.

Nevertheless, archiving the memories does not mean that they don't exist. The fact that they have been put on the shelf does not mean that they are not there, festering beneath the surface. So, while you are going about your day to day life, you may not experience any ill feelings. Yet, there are moments when certain triggers bring up such emotions. When this happens, your body's stress levels may begin to rise, along with other symptoms such as anxiety. Underlying, subconscious causes may also lead to depression.

A qualified hypnotist is unable to use hypnotic techniques in order to access your subconscious. When this happens, you are able to express your feelings and reveal what is truly affecting you. The way that a hypnotherapist gets you into a "trance" is through the use of a combination of relaxation and suggestion. There are no gimmicks or tricks like in the movies.

In essence, hypnosis is a state of deep relaxation in which your conscious mind shuts off. This enables the subconscious mind to emerge. At this point, the hypnotherapist would be able to determine what issues may be affecting you. At that point, you can begin addressing them through the conscious mind.

However, there is a caveat: when buried feelings begin to emerge, you must have proper counseling and support. The reason for this is that you may not be able to cope with these feelings on your own. As such, you will need to count with professional help so you can process such feelings and learn to manage them.

The biggest benefit of this course of action is that you will be able to identify what is affecting you. Therefore, you will be able to deal with these feelings and the corresponding physical symptoms which may be leading you to struggle with your weight. Most importantly, you will be able to heal emotional blockages which may have been lodged there for years.

Frequently taken medications for treating migraines, blood pressure, seizures, and depression, when used in excessive amounts—more than prescribed by your doctor—can lead to weight loss in addition to various other physical and mental health issues.

Stress is an emotion alters our body chemistry, and this changes our eating habits. When our bodies are under stress, more hormones are produced. These hormones depend on the degree of stress you have. In acute stress, your body releases epinephrine, whereas, in chronic stress, it releases corticotrophin.

Acute stress can be experienced in situations that are very dangerous, while chronic stress may occur in situations like separation, mourning, or anxiety. Stress can as well stop the body from releasing important hormones and at the same time, stimulate it to release others. When our bodies release cortisol and epinephrine in excess, it is a signal for preparing the body for action. These hormones push our system to get ready to handle a difficult situation or to run away from it as it is beyond our capability. Either of the above reactions could keep you alive or diminish the threat. Our emotions are affected by our brain and body, and at the same time, our brain and body affect our emotions.

For instance, when cortisol is released in excess, it affects metabolism. Energy is directed to our major parts of the body to prepare them for action. I know we have all been in a do or die situation, and we can all remember the energy we felt in our bodies; your heartbeat also increased, but the adrenaline did not last.

Our systems have a feedback cycle such that when the emergency is handled, the body starts releasing cortisol at its normal rate. This system is also influential to cortisol itself as it self-shuts itself. When cortisol goes to the brain, it gives it a command to stop the body from producing more of it. In the case of chronic stress, the system runs throughout, and it does not shut.

You find the production of cortisol keeps continuing and this makes us feel anxious or depressed. In periods when we are stressed, the brain gives instructions to the body to release some chemicals to handle the stress.

These chemicals affect our emotion center of the brain. Other than the influences of the brain chemicals on our emotions, other physiological influences alter our emotions.

These influences are the nutrients we get from food and access to fat deposits by the body. It is made possible by the location of the liver making it get abdominal fat and break it down to produce energy.

Nevertheless, when you have chronic stress, it is not easy to break down those fats quickly and at the same time, replace what is being used.

Therefore, the body tends to look for a quick replacement in fatty and sugary foods.

They replace the exhausted energy reserves and also comfort our emotions because of their high palatability.

These fatty foods may reduce stress in some of us, but when we over-consume them, we become obese. The psychological characteristics that help you to choose the comfort food of your choice are depression, neuroticism, premenstrual dysphoria, and sufferers of emotional eating. We can also note that the size of our meals and the content in it depend on the consumer's needs, expectations, and habits.

In regards to our discussion above, we have noted that what we eat is determined by neurotransmitters and hormones.

We can get different habits, depending on the degree of stress.

We eat food to replace the exhausted energy reserves due to chronic stress. Different individuals react differently to stress. For instance, one study by Oliver showed us that stress did not change the food quantity the participants consumed but that the participants with emotional eating disorders ate more of the comfort foods than those without stress or the eating disorder.

If our immediate response to the body demands during stressing periods were food, we would not be having so many cases of obesity. The problem lies in the type of food we run to consume to comfort us. Most obese and overweight people prefer foods that contribute to their conditions.

Therefore, food reduces stress, and it also produces it due to psychological and physiological problems. Different studies have found that some people select food because of their chemical effects, while others choose to meet their emotional needs as a response to stress. Emotional eaters eat more fatty, salty, or sugary foods as opposed to the belief that they eat food in large quantities. Finally, the relation between food and emotion is demonstrated well in a stressful situation. Stress has the power to alter our eating habits.

Just like in the case of weight, stress, and anxiety can induce in you weird eating habits that include overeating and under-eating.

This happens when you do not find an effective way of dealing with stress. Constantly eating because you are stressed has the same effect as alcohol. You will eat all you want, but when the food is digested and assimilated, your stress or anxiety will come back, maybe with an even higher intensity.

The food you eat because you think it will reduce stress is not normally healthy and balanced. A careful observation of such eating habits shows the kind of food that is eaten by the individual is mostly junk food, and the eating itself is irregular.

The other aspect of eating habits related to stress is eating less than the recommended amount or starving yourself. This is already a disaster before arrival. This is not only bad for your body health; it can also worsen your stress and anxiety level. Either way, you will always be alternating between a starvation/binge eating and stress.

During the fight/flight response, which is activated by adrenaline in the event of a threat or danger, we tend to get active and fidgety. Anxiety kicks in, and you feel wired-up as adrenaline responds to the threat of stress.

You find that you feel unsettled, and you may begin to run around anxiously, reaching out for a solution. Such anxiety triggers emotional eating. In an attempt to calm down, you find yourself eating or overeating unhealthy foods. This is a prevalent response to stress.

Anxiety makes you eat mindlessly, and you find yourself eating more without getting satisfied. You cannot even tell how much you have eaten because you are busy churning worrisome and stressful thoughts around your head, to the point where you cannot even focus on the taste of your food.

You eat more emotionally, and less mindfully when you are anxious and stressed, and you feel less satisfied, however more you may eat. This emotional and anxious overeating leads to weight gain.

Anxiety and stress can make someone engage in binge eating. One may go through a stressful event like losing a loved one or losing all his/her property and results in binge eating. Eating emotionally is not permanent, and it may, at times, not be binge eating.

A person who is anxious about a particular event or situation may result in binge eating. People who are anxious or stressed about something are more likely to binge eat. Binge eating can be caused by a stressful ordeal or a situation that makes one be anxious.

Relaxation Scripts

The art of relaxation is a state of mind. In other, you need to set your thoughts in such a way that leisure is essential. Even when you are eating, you can`t just keep consuming all the time.

You need to relax and take some break that will help your mind settle and think of other things.

The minds also need to shift from one aspect to the other. In other words, if you keep doing something for long, there are chances that you will get bored and hate it. In the same way, you can`t eat for more than an hour and expect that all is well. Even your jaws, let alone your teeth need to relax and prepare for another meal.

Also, if the snack is so sweet, there are chances that you can`t take all the time and eat everything at a go. You need to relax and allow the process of digestions to swallow, let alone.

Several studies have been carried out to determine the effects of failing to relax while eating. It is worth noting that if you eat without allowing your gut to shallow well, there are chances that you will be choked.

There are other cases where one fails to register in the brain that one is full since they are not relaxing. In other words, if your minds do not have time to relax, there are some complications that one may develop. For instance, people who develop the disorder of binge eating do not improve the condition in a single day.

However, it occurs gradually such that the minds fail to register that one is full. The desire to keep eating develops, and one thinks of eating rather than deducing anything else. They are the kind of people who will prefer eating at night, during the day and at any time. The art of eating in such a manner is not right as the mind does not relax.

One of the primary reasons that cause the brain or rather the body to develop the urge of relaxation is the fact that when one relaxes, there are several cells that rejuvenate, and one gains more energy from the tasks ahead of them.

One of the best methods that individuals prefer relaxing with is sleeping. After toiling for several hours, preferably after eating, a lot of people prefer sleeping so as they can relax. In other cases, it may lie down on a mat and reflect on what has been going on.

The art of relaxing is essential in the sense that it allows one to have some more time to think of the things that can be done for life or rather the eating habits. Relaxation is essential as one will have some ample time to analyze whether the food is taken or the activities being done were achieved in the right way.

The other aspect that people consider as a means of relaxing exercises. After having a heavy meal, the best means of relaxing is taking a ball or any other item that will help you do some exercise. It is worth noting that when you exercise, the body graves for more energy. In other words, your body will require more energy to sustain the exercises.

Thus, the food taken will be broken down quickly, and you will have more reasons for eating again after a period of six to eight hours.

Scholars have identified that people who can exercise from time to time have some of the nest digestion processes. In other words, there are not affected by issues of digestion or rather complications that develop from improper digestion. The food they take is well broken down and converted into energy that is required in the exercises.

Mind games are the best means of relaxing after a heavy meal. Although some snacks encourage one to sleep, a mind game plays a critical role in ensuring that all the food is broken down quickly.

It is worth noting that the brain uses a lot of energy to deliberate in a task.

For instance, when you are playing a game such as chess, you will be required to think and think well. It is worth noting that when you are considering as such, the energy consumed is more than the power you would use to lift a certain weight deliberately. Therefore, a mind game will play a critical role in allowing your mind or rather your body to relax and regain the strength of doing other activities. In other words, even after eating, the body requires some time to relax. Relaxation helps the cell as well as the tissues of an individual to regain some aspects of healing for the future.

For instance, if one has been eating, there are chances that there were some cells destroyed in the mouth, let alone the alimentary canal. One may require some more time to heal and regain the strength of eating again.

Relaxation is essential.

The how and the, when to relax, depends on the type of food taken or the activity that one was engaged with previously. For instance, if you have been doing some hard labor, there are cases where you might feel that you need to lie down and relax.

In addition, if you have been sitting down for long, there are chances that you will need some exercises to help you relax. The aspect is linked to the fact that when you stretch, you allow your cells to relax and prepare for the next activity or instead of the other session. Also, if you have been sitting in a class for long, there are chances that your body needs some time to relax. In such a situation, after eating, the best method of relaxing is engaging in one exercise.

The aspect is critical in the sense that you will have time to stretch and regain some of the energy loss when you are sited. He minds to regain its strength, and you will be in a good position to grasp more of what your teacher is saying.

People react differently to hypnosis. Some are able to continue a conversation while hypnotized. Some people feel a complete sense of detachment from their surroundings. Others experience a heightened sense of relaxation which removes all stress. Whereas, other people have described their state of mind as feeling outside their conscious choice, giving them a feeling of complete control from their hypnotist.

Only 10% of adults are difficult to hypnotize and if you are a person who loves to fantasize and have a vivid imagination, you will do well.

Hilgard is a well-known theory. Hilgard's neodissociation theory suggests that people in a hypnotic state experience a split consciousness. One mental stream of activity focuses on suggestion and the other gathers information outside of your conscious awareness.

There are common myths about hypnotism I would like to discredit, these are simply untrue. The first myth is the one that is most common. The myth claims that you will have no memory of your hypnotized state. This myth blows things out of proportion because amnesia only occurs in rare cases. Then there is posthypnotic amnesia which is a temporary state. Posthypnotic amnesia can make you forget things that happened just before or after hypnosis.

Your memory will come back. Don't allow this to deter you. Another common myth says that you can be hypnotized against your will. This is a blatant lie. An untruth that was made famous by movies and fiction. The myth where people lose control is another myth I would like to tell you about. Remember there is a difference between hypnosis and mentalism. Hypnotism requires you to participate willingly.

You are in constant control during a hypnosis session. So please don't believe any of these myths (Cherry, 2019).

I would like to focus on using combined techniques for hypnosis for this audio guide. One of these techniques is solution-focused hypnotherapy (SFH). This form of hypnotherapy is a combined effort between the hypnotist and yourself. I find it easier to work toward a solution rather than running away from a problem.

Set yourself a goal and take small steps forward. Don't crucify yourself for being a smoker. Instead, use hypnosis to become a non-smoker with time and effort. Another technique is behavioral hypnotherapy. This form of hypnosis is used to modify future behavior and habits. Hypnosis bypasses your conscious mind and allows you to speak to your subconscious mind directly.

Changing behavior is like planting a seed.

The deeper the inception goes, the more likely it is to stick and grow. And last but not least, I will use inspiration from cognitive hypnotherapy as well. Cognitive hypnotherapy focuses on the thoughts and emotions attached to certain behavior.

I will approach hypnosis using a combination of these three techniques. Behavioral hypnotherapy will focus on your behavior but you will benefit from understanding the emotion attached to that behavior through cognitive hypnotherapy. Using these two techniques combined with solution-focused hypnotherapy allow you to see your end goal and strive for it (Fulcher, 2018).

Now that you understand hypnosis better, I want you to understand the benefits of hypnosis. Let's look at a few examples of how hypnosis can help you.

Fear or phobia has a debilitating effect on your mind and body and hypnosis can help you overcome your fear. Fear plays a major role in your approach to social experiences or trying something new. Your fear affects your confidence when approaching a new person or when you have to get up on stage. Stage fright is definitely a form of fear. Fear also holds you back from skydiving for the first time because you over-analyze the possible outcomes. Thinking about everything that can go wrong before you jump. Being afraid of public speaking can affect your chances of acing your job interview too.

Another great advantage of hypnotism is to quit an addiction. People who want to quit smoking are the most frequent newcomers to the world of hypnotism. Add hypnotherapy to your current methods of trying to quit. As a matter of fact, it is advised by the National Center for Complementary and Integrative Health.

Hypnosis is also a great approach to anxiety and stress. Stress and anxiety can affect you physically and mentally. They can break you down and weaken your mind. A weakened mind is vulnerable to future stress and anxiety. Being anxious will prevent you from living the life you want to. Let's help you live the life you deserve (Russel, 2018).

Another key benefit of hypnosis is deep sleep. Deep sleep is essential to your mind's well-being. Without enough deep sleep, your brain struggles to function. Insomnia is not only defined as the loss of sleep but it's also defined as the loss of sleep quality. Millions of people are affected by insomnia worldwide. To combat this problem through hypnosis, we need to understand what deep sleep is.

There are two main categories of sleep. One is called rapid eye movement (REM), the other is called non-REM sleep. Your body and mind cycles through both stages in a regular pattern when you sleep. You will cycle through these stages a few times in a single night. Hypnosis will teach you to regulate this pattern so you can achieve more deep sleep. Deep sleep helps your brain recover from thinking and is essential to your mind's health. Deep sleep encourages your pituitary glands to secrete human growth hormones to help tissues in your body grow and regenerate. This leaves you feeling refreshed when you wake up.

A mind that doesn't gain enough deep sleep in one day, will compensate the next day by cycling through your sleep pattern rapidly. This will deprive your brain of the stable pattern your mind needs. Your brain will find it difficult to store memories and retain information. Hypnosis can increase the amount of time you spend in deep sleep by 80%. Deep sleep is also called slow-wave sleep (Mozes, 2014).

You feel another gentle, warm touch on your skin. Trust my voice and don't be afraid. Keep breathing deeply in through your nose and slowly out through your pursed lips. Blow the air out gently each time. Listen to your heart beating. One, two three, four, and five. Feel yourself soaking up the sunlight. Each ray touching your skin is more gentle, more calm. Each ray, a perfect amount of warm.

Notice how calm you are. No wind is blowing, only your breath. The soft, gentle sand kissing your skin from beneath. The warm, refreshing water tickling your toes from the sea. The sun dancing warmly off your skin from above. Count with me in your mind. One, two, three, four, and five. Every number is two heartbeats. Breathe in deeply with every two beats and breathe out slowly with another two beats. Feel your mind transcend further into relaxation. You are so comfortable, more comfortable than you have ever been before.

Keep your focus on my voice. Remember to feel every beat of your heart pumping relaxation through your veins. Breathe in through your nose and out through your mouth, slowly. You can see something now but you are unsure what you see.

Notice how your heart keeps the gentle rhythm as you look closer at this unknown image you see. Every word is spoken, transcends you deeper. You are so comfortable and calm. Fear has no place anymore.

This unknown image beckons you, closer and closer. You feel drawn to the unknown image in a welcoming way. Listen to your heartbeat. One, two, three, four, and five. Breathe deeply through your nose and hold your breath for a moment. Count to three and release your breath slowly.

Remember to purse your lips lightly as you do so.

Sleep Scripts

In order to properly set yourself up for a meditation experience, you need to make sure that you have a quiet space where you can engage in your meditation. You want to be as uninterrupted as possible so that you do not stir awake from your meditation session. Aside from having a quiet space, you should also make sure that you are comfortable in the space that you will be in.

For some of the meditations, I will share, you can be lying down or doing this meditation before bed so that the information sinks in as you sleep. For others, you are going to want to be sitting upright, ideally with your legs crossed on the floor, or with your feet planted on the floor as you sit in a chair.

Staying in a sitting position, especially during morning meditations, will help you stay awake and increase your motivation. Laying down during these meditations earlier in the day may result in you draining your energy and feeling completely exhausted, rather than motivated. As a result, you may actually work against what you are trying to achieve.

Each of these meditations is going to involve a visualization practice; however, if you find that visualization is generally difficult for you, you can simply listen. The key here is to make sure that you keep as open of a mind as possible so that you can stay receptive to the information coming through these guided meditations.

Aside from all of the above, listening to low music, using a pillow or a small blanket, and dressing in comfortable loose clothing will all help you have better meditations. You want to make sure that you make these experiences the best possible so that you look forward to them and regularly engage in them. As well, the more relaxed and comfortable you are, the more receptive you will be to the information being provided to you within each meditation.

This is a great meditation to engage in during the day anywhere from one to three times per week, or at bedtime.

They say that meditating right before you fall asleep can be particularly potent, as you are meditating during a time where your subconscious mind is particularly active, and your conscious mind is already beginning to fall asleep. During this time, you are most likely to experience the level of relaxation and receptivity that is needed for your subconscious mind to really digest the changes that you are seeking to make within it.

"You'll fall into a deep sleep soon". I am sure you have heard this famous phrase. Well, Bonnie has. She considered hypnosis something mysterious or half-serious and a half-spiritual ritual that she had absolutely no intention of trying. She hadn't even believed that her problem had roots in her subconscious.

It was Evelin who convinced her about the benefits of this practice after an incredible change in her. One day she met one of her ex-dates from the past before her marriage, George who had become a famous therapist and offered some free sessions to her for old times' sake.

Evelin talked about her marriage, her divorce and how

she let herself go. George proposed hypnotherapy to reveal the underlying problems and ultimately induce her subconscious toward wanting to be beautiful again and losing weight. After some months of hard work, Evelin started to change. She became braver and more confident. She became wonderful. It was about her radiance in the beginning.

It was like she started knowing who was she in reality and it gave her spirit. After a short time, she began experiencing another benefit as well: she lost weight (and gained love). She lost a lot of weight. She returned to her pre-divorce shape.

As a good mother, she wanted the same happy results for her daughter, but first, she had to overcome Bonnie's skepticism about hypnosis. That's why it was necessary to make some notes about the material, as we will do in this part of the book.

When we are asleep, the brain waves slow down and produce the so-called delta frequency waves. When it reveals relatively higher frequency vigilance, this is called beta frequency waves. Research has shown that brain waves are at theta frequency during hypnosis. In the theta frequency, there is both a level of subconscious awareness as well as a high concentration in sleep.

It has been noticed that theta frequency occurs more frequently in the brains of people who are more susceptible to hypnosis. Besides, some researchers claim that hypnotizability is inherited and strongly conditioned by the presence of specific genes (Adachi, Jensen, Lee, Miró, Osman, Tomé-Pires, 2016).

Sleep induction isn't a truth serum in the real world. Even though during subliminal therapy, you are progressively open to a recommendation, regardless, you have through and through freedom and good judgment. Nobody can make you state anything you would prefer not to say — lie or not.

In a word, the genuine brains behind the strategy are your subliminal personality—it does the greater part of your reasoning, and it settles on a ton of choices about what you are doing. Your cognizant personality works when you're conscious of evaluating a great deal of these considerations, settling on decisions, and setting a few thoughts in motion. It likewise procedures and transfers crisp information to the subliminal personality. In any case, the cognizant personality escapes the way when you're sleeping, and your subliminal has a free rule.

Specialists pose that sleep induction's significant unwinding and focusing activities capacity to quiet and quell the cognizant personality to take a less dynamic part in your procedure of reasoning. You are as yet mindful of what is happening in this state. However, your cognizant personality takes your intuitive personality rearward sitting arrangement. This empowers you and the subliminal specialist to work with the intuitive legitimately. It seems as though the technique for trancelike influence is opening up a control board inside your mind.

Insomnia can result from stress, poor eating habits, and bad sleeping habits. When it occurs, you might have difficulties sleeping at night, waking up in the middle of the night, feeling sleepy during the day, or lack of concentration.

You find that the main reason an individual lacks sleep is due to some mental and emotional issues that they are going through. When it occurs, it results in a lot of anxiety, depression, or stress. All these are mental issues that can be controlled by having a change of mindset. As you meditate, you analyze the various challenges that you are going through.

In that process, you realize the causes of the challenges and the effects that they have on your mental wellbeing. At the same time, you can come up with some possible solutions to the problem at hand.

When you adopt a routine of regularly meditating, you will realize a lot of change in your sleep life. You will find it easier to rest since your mind is at peace, and it helps you in overcoming stress.

Chapter 7.   Bedtime Meditations For Kids

The following are sample meditation scripts that you can teach your kids.

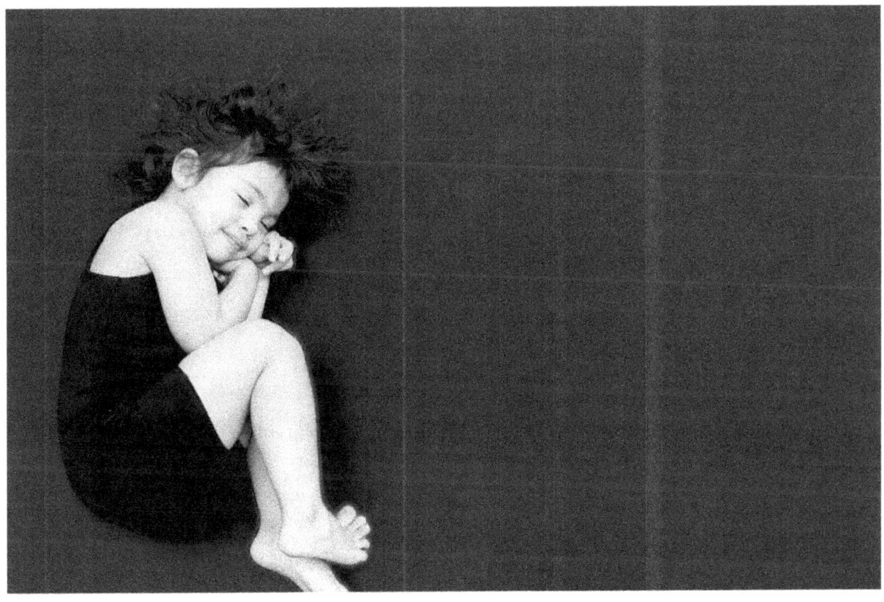

The Relaxing Warm Water

Start by finding a position that you are comfortable in, and of course, your favorite couch or chair in your house. Make sure that your chair or couch is big enough to allow you to sit down with your legs crossed and that it has a soft and fluffy cushion so you will not feel any discomfort later.

Take three long breaths and as you are breathing, imagine that relaxation and comfort is slowly flowing towards you, like warm water slowly hugging your body and then entering you so you feel warm and comfortable inside too. Begin with your eyelids, try to feel the pleasant warm water pressing against it, and imagine that it is slowly climbing up to your forehead. Now, it flows up into your head and covers your hair, then, it falls at the back of your neck and as it touches it, your neck begins to start relaxing.

The relaxing warm water is now flowing down your face, making your cheeks a bit warm and loosening your jaw. Your teeth are unclenched, and all of the muscles in your head and neck are relaxed. If you find the water to be a bit heavy on top of your head, imagine moving it further down to your shoulders or wherever you want it to be so long as you feel comfortable. Let the warm, relaxing water flow down from your shoulders and in to your arms. As it touches your shoulders and arms, the muscles start to loosen up and you feel as if your arms are floating in water. They are light and do not drag down your shoulders.

The water flows all the way down, hugging your elbows, and then your hands. It reaches your fingers and wraps your fingertips in its warmth and comfort. Each of your fingers are feeling warm, and the water is slipping in between. Your fingers become submerged in it, and the warmth embraces each one of them.

Any tension that you feel in your arms, your shoulder, your neck, head, and fingers start melting away. The melting tension turns into mist and floats away from your body. The muscles in your back, your spine, and your tailbone, start to unclench as the warm water embraces them. The warm water flows along both sides of your spine like a stream and makes a warm puddle at your tailbone. Your body can now sink a little bit more into the chair, into the puddle of warm water that has covered you in a warm, relaxing hug.

Your chest and stomach area are loosening up, and your breathing starts slowing down as you feel the warmth creep inside your chest. You begin to feel very comfortable as the warmth travels down to your stomach and rests there, like your favorite hot drink. After it settles in your stomach, it then flows further down, wrapping your thighs, your knees, and then your lower legs and feet. The warmth creeps in between your toes. You begin to feel that even the smallest muscles in your feet are slowly relaxing, as if the water was massaging your soles.

Your feet feel as if you have worn a pair of very tight shoes all day long, and you have just removed those shoes and dipped your feet into warm water. Every breath you slowly take, in, out, in, out, makes you feel more and more relaxed. All the tension in your legs are being pushed down to the soles of your feet every time you inhale, and every time you exhale, the remaining tension comes out of your mouth or nose as warm mist.

After freeing your entire body from all the tension that it had, imagine that you are slowly standing up from the couch and walking towards your door. You feel very light, as if your entire body has just been thoroughly massaged and you have bathed in a warm bathtub for a long time. As you open the door, instead of seeing the usual place outside your house, you are now transported to a beautiful beach.

The sun is shining brightly but it does not feel hot. You can feel the cool breeze caressing your entire body, the sand under your toes softly embraces them, you can hear the ocean waves or the calls of your favorite birds in the beach, and you can smell the salty smell of the sea in the air. You could be alone in this beach, or if you want, you could also be with your favorite friends, siblings, parents, cousins, or neighbors. You can also add any animal that you want to add and imagine them laying around the sand, enjoying the warm sunlight and the cool sea breeze. The sea can be either wavy or very, very calm, like a sheet of metal reflecting the sun. Today is the most perfect day to be outside in the beach.

Find a place in the beach where you feel most comfortable in and sit down and rest. You can sit or lay down in the sand, and nothing in the world can affect you. You have left your problems behind. No one can disturb you here, and everyone that are present in the beach are people that you love to be around with. Your place in the beach is very peaceful and very comfortable. You feel the sand as you sit or lie down, and the warmth from the sun is hugging you very gently. The sound of the waves and the birds lightly fill your ears as you slowly close your eyes and let the relaxation and comfort embrace you.

Inside you, the warmth from the sun starts to glow out,

and you feel that your skin is slowly warming up from the inside. Your chest, your stomach, your legs, and your back are slowly coated in warm sunlight both inside and outside, and your head is light, as if it is a cloud floating the sky. The warmth from inside slowly spreads out to your arms, legs fingertips, toes, and even to the tips of your ears and hair. You notice that the palms of your hands are becoming warmer, like you have just been holding a warm bowl with your favorite soup in it. Allow this warmth to stay and flow throughout your body as you listen to the pleasant ocean waves and feel the cool sea breeze lightly touching your skin.

After a moment, we start traveling back home. Imagine yourself slowly standing u p and opening your eyes, then following the path that you walked before to get to your house's door. As you open the door, imagine yourself smiling and returning to your couch where you were sitting or lying down, and very gently, open your eyes. Count slowly from 1 to 10 as you look at the room and take a deep breath and exhale.

An Adventure in Ice Cream World

Find somewhere you can sit comfortably in. Slowly close your eyes and take a deep breath and exhale very slowly. Do these five times with your eyes still closed. Today, you will be going to a palace made of your favorite delicious ice cream, chocolates, cakes, and candies.

Imagine standing up and walking outside your house. Outside, you see a lot of hills, but instead of grass, the hills are coated with your favorite flavor of ice cream. The hills are like giant scoops of that ice cream, and you rush towards them. You take off your shoes or slippers and you feel the ground. It is fluffy and a bit cold but the cold does not hurt your feet. The smell of your favorite ice cream flavor covers the air, and the sunlight is very bright but not hot at all.

You dig your hands in the ice cream ground, and you take a bite, tasting that very delicious and cool flavor. After one bite however, you hear the sound of a stream. When you look down form where you are standing, you see that the stream is made up of warm melted chocolate. You take a deep breath, you close your eyes, and you slide down the ice cream hill.

At the stream, you smell the rich chocolatey air and you

dip one finger into the stream. The melted chocolate is warm, and it tastes like your favorite chocolate in the entire world. You see your favorite cup beside your feet, and you pick it up, then dip it into the chocolate river. You close your eyes and take in the rich smell of the chocolate. You breathe in and out and relax yourself, before taking a sip of the drink. A cold wind blows under you and your feet are suddenly feeling cold. You dip them into the warm melted chocolate stream and you instantly feel much better. You leave your feet in the stream, relaxing in the warmth, and lay back while closing your eyes, enjoying the feel of gentle sunlight and a cool breeze touching your skin. The smell of your favorite ice cream flavor and your favorite chocolate fill the air, and you smile while laying back and warming up your feet in the stream.

After taking five deep breaths, slowly inhaling the pleasant-smelling air and very gently exhaling it from your mouth, imagine that you are now standing up. The warm chocolate is slowly melting away from your feet, and every time you take a step, you leave behind a chocolate footprint on the ice cream ground. After you walk for a bit, you see your favorite snow pants hanging on a tree, but the tree does not have leaves. Instead, it is covered with all of the candies that you like most in the world. You take the snow pants and wear it. It feels very warm and you feel the muscles in your legs relax when they touch the fabric of the pants.

Up another hill, you see a banana boat, and a gentle slope. You feel excited, as you run towards the boat and find a comfortable seat. As you sit inside the boat, you notice that the boat inside is very pleasantly warm and comfortable, and your lower body slowly relaxes as if you were sitting in a bathtub filled halfway with warm water. You gently close your eyes, breathe in through your nose, and out again in your nose. You do this very slowly five more times. You then imagine opening your eyes and seeing the thrilling slope that will surely give you a fantastic ride. At the bottom where you will land, the ground is made up of giant soft fluffy marshmallows.

You put your hands at each side of your hips, and very slowly, you begin to push towards the boat towards the slope. You whoosh past everything, making all the ice cream hills and candy trees disappear in a blur, and you laugh as the cool air hits your face and sends your hair back. The bottom is still a bit far so you close your eyes and you smile a very wide smile. You feel the air going into your mouth and you try to inhale it. The air mixes with the butterflies in your stomach and you feel giddy and very happy. When you open your eyes, you see that the giant marshmallows are already coming closer and closer. When the boat hit the marshmallow, you get thrown off and you bounce in the marshmallow. You feel exhilarated. That was such an exciting slide.

You smile widely and you take in slow breaths as you lie down on the soft fluffy marshmallows. You close your eyes and you feel your back and your shoulders sink a bit into the marshmallow like they would when you lie down in a very fluffy bed. The marshmallows begin to massage your shoulder and back and you feel the muscles in there just untangling. All the tension in your muscles are slowly disappearing as your back and shoulders are being massaged by the marshmallows. You feel very comfortable and relaxed.

After a while, you open your eyes and stand up. You walk past the soft marshmallows and you head towards a field made of very powdery snow. When you come near, you realize that the snow smells like your favorite cereal, so you taste a little bit and are very surprised. The snow looks like snow but it is very tasty. You smile and you lie down in order to make a snow angel. You close your eyes and take a refreshing breath through your nose. The air smells like your favorite cereal, and you breathe out through your nose. You do these five more times, and each time you do this, you flap your arms and legs to slowly make a snow angel.

Afterwards, you start to feel a bit cold, so you stand up and see a coat made of waffles in the ground. When you wear it, it instantly warms your entire body, and you feel a warm, calming sensation in your chest, shoulders, and arms. After feeling the warmth slowly spread throughout your body, you hear a laughter at the distance. You run towards the sound and find a laughing child and your favorite animal tossing snowballs at each other. They call you to come play with them, and you quickly run towards them. You form a very big snowball and you hit the child, but after the child trips down, you then get hit by a snowball made by your favorite animal and all of you laugh.

Afterwards, you look up to the sky and see snowflakes made of different gems and metal. Some were golden in color, others were made of diamonds, and some were all sorts of colors that you could think of. All three of you decide to pick your favorite color among the falling snowflakes. After a while, you notice that the sun is already setting, and that it was slowly getting colder.

Your neck feels especially cold, so your friends quickly knit up a scarf made from your favorite snowflakes and it warms up your neck very well. You close your eyes and breathe slowly, feeling the warmth hugging your neck and spreading upwards to your head and to the tip of your ears. Your friends also made themselves their own scarves and you all stand in comfortable warmth.

Later, you notice a bright orange glow not far from where you are standing. You go there and find a fire that was warm but never hot. You try to come closer to see if it would get hot, but it never did. It was just a pleasant orange warmth. You slowly poked a finger to the fire and was surprised to notice that the fire did not burn at all. All three of you decided to sit down around the fire and place your hands inside it. It was very warm and very relaxing, and the fire changed color depending on what you wanted it to be. The fire slowly creeps up your clothes, but it never burned. It just felt very warm, and it slowly covered you in a very cool looking bright fire that never burned your skin or your clothes. The fire also smelled like your favorite shampoo. You close your eyes and inhale the smell, and when you opened them, you found the door to your bedroom in front of you.

You slowly opened the door and you found yourself inside

your bedroom. The bed felt very inviting as you had such a long and fun day. You laid down your bed. Slowly, you take in five breaths and you very gently open your eyes to find yourself back in the real world. You feel every part of your body relax and you take one last deep breath before standing up with a smile from all the fun you experienced.

A Script for Exams

Find a place in your house or anywhere else where you can freely be alone. The place should ideally be quiet and free from as much clutter as possible. Find a spot where you can sit down with your legs crossed. Try to bring a cushion so you will be more comfortable as you sit. If you are doing this in your room, try to clean your room first by putting everything in place. Your goal should be to have as much space and as few distractions as possible.

As you sit down, slowly close your eyes and try to imagine that all your weight is concentrated in a ball somewhere inside your abdomen. Imagine that the weight of your head is slowly melting down to your shoulders, and that in turn melts down to your chest until all these collects and forms a heavy ball at the center of your abdomen. Focus your mind on that particular center. As you imagine this, breathe slowly and allow your hands to gently fall in place on top of your lap. Try to imagine that all the weight from your shoulder, arms, and head have all been transferred to that center, and all that is left is lightness.

Take a moment to pat yourself in the back. You are doing this because you are dedicated, you have a goal, and you are committed to do whatever it takes to reach that. Thank yourself for being strong enough to not turn away from the stress that you are feeling. Congratulate yourself that you are trying your best to face that. It might be that you are struggling to concentrate for your studies, or you are simply overwhelmed by everything that you have to memorize and learn for your exam. It might be that you are feeling pressured to get a high score, or to simply not fail. Whatever your reason maybe, do not worry. You are here, you are doing something to help you achieve your goal, and that is all that matters.

Through your nose, inhale very slowly, hold your breath for five seconds, and slowly exhale though your mouth. Do these five more times as you repeat these words inside your head: "I will succeed. This stress will soon go away". Feel each breath as the air passes through you.

Every breath that you take places you more firmly into the floor. You are becoming more stable. You are becoming safer. Nothing can harm you. Nothing can scare you. You will succeed.

Acknowledge your own presence. Feel the air that is passing through you. You are making the air pass through you. You are here. You are being committed. You are being strong. You are not the problem. The problem is the way you look at your studying, at the way you look at your exam. But you can change this. You will change this.

Imagine a cactus in front of you. Try to visualize what a cactus looks like for you. How big is it? Does it have a flower? What is its color? How spiky is it? Are the spikes thin or thick? Try to fill in as much details as you can on the cactus. Engage all of your senses in recreating it inside your head. When you put your nose close to it, does it smell nice? Think of all these sensations and relate it to the cactus. Visualize your own interactions with it. Imagine touching it. How does it feel? It hurts, right?

Now, gently shift your focus from the cactus to yourself. Imagine that the cactus is slowly floating away, and in front of you, you see yourself. What do you look like? Recreate your entire body inside your mind with as much details as you can. What is the color of your hair? What about your eyes? Can you try counting how many teeth you can see when you smile? How do you think do you smell like? Do you have any scars or birthmarks on your body? Try looking at them intently.

Imagine that you can see your eyes are projecting all of y our thoughts and worries like a movie. Can you see yourself stressing over the exam? Now try to look at the background of that movie. You see other people, right? You see classmates, you see other students, you even see your teachers and your parents. You are not alone in this movie, right?

Blur out yourself from the movie and slowly focus on the people at the background. What do you think is your seatmate thinking about? Try to picture him/her out inside your head and see whether or not he/she is feeling stressed about the exam too. What can you possible say to him/her to lessen that stress?

Continue breathing, taking in air very slowly and exhaling it through your mouth. You see, you are not alone in the movie. You are not alone in this exam, and you are not the only student in the world that is feeling stressed right now because of it.

Breathe in through your nose. Hold your breath for eight seconds. Exhale through your mouth very slowly. Imagine that every breath you take adds confidence to yourself. Now, imagine that every breath you exhale adds confidence to others: to your classmates, friends, and all the other students in the world that are feeling stressed right now for the exam. Imagine that every time you breathe, your body becomes lighter and lighter. The heavy ball at the center of your stomach is slowly melting through your skin and evaporating like mist. You are not alone in this. You will succeed.

Now visualize that you are back inside your classroom and your test paper is already in your desk. Take a deep breath, exhale, and slowly run your hands over the sheet of paper. This exam is just a sheet of paper. Imagine picking it up and letting a strong breeze carry it away. A light, sheet of paper. You are not alone. You are safe. You can succeed in this.

Gently open your eyes. Take a deep breath, and slowly stand up.

A Flower in the Mud

Imagine that you are a flower. Try to visualize your favorite type of flower. What color is it? How does it smell like? Imagine that you are this flower. Your feet are slowly growing roots. You are stuck firmly in the ground, and nothing can pull you out. Imagine the feeling of mud as it slowly rises up, first up to your knees, and later up to your neck. When you look up, you see the sky.

The sun is shining very brightly, but it is not hot. You feel the cool breeze gently touching your face. But your body cannot move. You are stuck inside this pool of mud. You want to rise above this mud. You want your body and not just your face to feel the cool breeze, to feel the warmth of the bright sun. You want to grow up, up above all this mud, and bask under the warmth and the breeze.

Slowly, imagine that your roots are spreading outwards, digging even deeper into the earth. Take a deep breath. Slowly take in air through your nose and exhale it through your mouth. Every time you inhale, imagine that your roots are taking in nutrients from the earth. The nutrients flow from the base of your feet up towards your head. It feels like being dipped in a warm bath. The nutrients relax your muscles as it covers them with comfortable warmth.

Every time you exhale, imagine that your body, your stem, is slowly growing up. Your roots take in the nutrients as you inhale, and your body stretches past the mud as you exhale. Your stem grows taller and taller. The mud is now at your waist. Imagine waving your arms to the cool breeze. They are green leave. Your head is the flower. The warm sunlight is embracing the flower and its leaves. You breathe in and out again, each time you become taller and taller. Now, the mud is only up to your knees. Your waist feels the cool breeze and the warm sun, and you gently smile as every breath bring in more nutrient for you to grow taller.

Now, you are standing above the mud. Your roots re still keeping you in place, but your entire body is already above ground. You sway with the gentle breeze and you tilt your head upwards, so your petals can catch the warmth of the sun. You are beautiful, colorful, fragrant, and free.

Imagine that people are passing by you, and every time they see you, they stop and marvel at how beautiful your petals are. Your determination to grow out of the mud made you free, made you experience the sun and the breeze, made everyone smile as they pass by you because they could not help it. You are standing tall. You are beautiful. You are determined. You have succeeded.

Very gently, you smile, then open your eyes.

General Muscle Relaxation Script

In this exercise, you will be tensing and relaxing the different muscle groups in your body in a systematic manner as you meditate. Try to find a place where you can be comfortable in, preferably somewhere quiet. With this exercise, you may choose to either open or close your eyes. Before doing this, try to tense up some of your muscles throughout your body. It can be your hands, or your arms, or the muscles in your stomach. Try to tense them and be aware of how it feels when they are fully tensed. Alternatively, you may also try to tense muscles but only very gently, just enough that you are feeling a slight tugging in them.

Start by taking deep, slow breaths. Pay attention to your breath as it flows from your nose down to your chest and finally in your abdomen. Let it sit there for five seconds, then very slowly, exhale through your mouth. As you do this, check-up on your current thoughts and emotional state. What is it that you are thinking most about today? What have you been feeling these past few days? Pay close attention to these things. Acknowledge that you are indeed thinking about them. Now, very gently, imagine that each time you exhale, one of these thoughts or emotions is being flushed out from your body. Do this until you can feel a comfortable silence in your mind. Your goal should be to only think about your breathing.

Next, slowly tense the muscles in your right forearm while making a fist with your right hand. Allow the rest of the arm to stay relaxed. Try doing this over and over until you can reach this balance. Feel the sensation of tensing your forearm and hand. Compare this feeling with the feeling of relaxation in your other arm, and throughout your body. Imagine that you are isolating all the tension in your body into just these muscles, leaving the rest of your body free and relaxed. When you feel that you are ready, inhale slowly through your nose, and exhale very gently through your mouth. As you exhale, imagine that the tension you built up in your right arm is slowly being released. Imagine the tension as water, and that every time you exhale, your arm is slowly leaking out this water until it is empty and relaxed. Pay attention to your now relaxed right arm. How does it feel now that it is free from so much tension? Repeat this entire process with your left forearm and fist. Do this again on any part of your body until you feel calm and relaxed.

Chapter 8.   Traits You Will Pick Up from Practicing Mindfulness Meditation

In addition to the numerous benefits of mindfulness meditation for your body and mind, there are various positive personality traits that you will pick up as your practice regularly and diligently. Let us look at some of these traits:

Living in the Moment

Living in the moment and fully immersed in the experience of life is the most wonderful trait you will develop with mindfulness meditation. The benefits of living in the moment are many including:

Having a rich life experience - Most of us are scared to let go of our thoughts and regrets from our past or our dreams for the future because there is a misconception that by doing so, we will become unemotional and, perhaps, an automaton instead of being human. The irony is this; when we live in the past or in the future, we leave a large part of our life experience in an unreal environment.

The only reality is the present moment and if we can put our entire body and mind in this present moment, then the emotional, spiritual, physical, and other human experiences become more powerful and richer than before. We end up leading a fuller life with mindfulness meditation than without it.

Focusing on the most important thing – By living in the moment, our energies are used in the most optimal way so that we can give our best and focus on the most important thing in our life; the present moment. What we do in the present decides our future. So, instead of living in a nebulous future, create a robust one by living fully in the tangible present.

Building better rapport – Living in the moment means you are completely connected with the people who are with you right now and right here. Your body and mind are focused on them which enhances the connection and rapport; the bedrock of any successful relationship. Being present in the moment means you are with your partner in mind and spirit, and paying attention to his or her every nuance of communication. Therefore, living in the moment helps you build strong and powerful relationships.

Mindfulness meditation helps you build and develop this crucial trait of living in the moment and leveraging its varied benefits that affect all aspects of your life positively.

Non-Judging

Being judgmental about everything and everyone around you results in plenty of needless hatred. Every time you feel, touch, see, hear, or sense anything, you are so habituated into deciding whether you like the sensation or not, that you are driven to form a judgment which, in turn, creates stress and anxiety. It is liberating to simply feel and sense life around you without judgment. Mindfulness meditation facilitates the building of a non-judgmental personality. The benefits are huge including:

It opens your body and mind to new experiences – Look back at your life and ask yourself how many times you have chosen to say no to things because you have formed a predetermined idea that you are 'not going to like it.' If you leave out judgment, you will see a rise in the number of new experiences that promise to bring you joy, pleasure, and happiness if you can avoid being foolishly blind.

Improved relationships with people – When you choose

not to judge and just be there for your friends and loved ones, the quality of your relationships and friendships will improve. People will open up with you knowing that you are not going to judge them, and they will confide in you without feeling guilty about their actions.

Your friends will be willing to share their deepest thoughts with you safe in the knowledge that you will not ridicule them. All this openness with people in your life will result in improved quality of relationships with enhanced intimacy, love, and affection.

Improved sense of spirituality – Being free of judgments liberates you and helps you become more spiritual and open to giving and receiving love from the divine and also from people around you. Your sense of compassion improves significantly and you will be able to forgive yourself and other people more easily than before resulting in your spirituality rising up a few notches.

Happy person – The liberation from the stress of having to label everything and everyone around as good, bad, average, right, wrong, or in any other way is so powerful that you become a happier person than when you were a judgmental individual. The complexities and complications of putting people and things in various predetermined places does not weigh you down anymore making you feel light, happy, and joyous.

Additionally, your ability to remain non-judgmental will free you of the burden associated with the worries of what other people think of you. You become resilient to criticism and take them constructively without getting emotionally attached. Instead, you use those criticisms wisely to improve yourself.

Understanding the Nature of Thought

Our thoughts flow like the wheel of an endlessly moving mill. Sometimes, we feel we can control our thoughts and sometimes, it seems impossible to control them. Sometimes, you seem to be able to discern between one thought and another, and sometimes, the thoughts seem to be like a big baggage of complexities thrown together with no order or rhythm.

Simply put, thoughts are like little conversations that go on endlessly in our heads. They are opinions, understandings, ideas, emotions, and everything else that keeps taking place in our heads with or without our knowledge. As we keep focusing on the flow of our thoughts during mindfulness meditation, we will slowly but surely develop the power to understand the true nature of our thoughts. We will be able to see how easy it is for our thoughts to control the way we behave because we will notice that our thoughts drive our emotions which, in turn, drive our actions.

As we progress in the intensity of our meditation, we will understand the true nature of thoughts and emotions. We will realize that our mind which forms these thoughts can be manipulated to form different thoughts for the same situation.

For example, if you have failed in an endeavor, the first instinctive thought would be related to emotions of sadness and regret for having failed. Your behavior will reflect these emotions, and you will begin to look for reasons to fail including finding people and things to blame.

However, if you paused for a little while, and took a couple of deep breaths, and directed your mind to think of the learning and knowledge you received from the failed endeavor or then the emotions will be quite different despite the situation not changing. This is only a small example of how powerful the mind is when it comes to directing our thoughts in the way we want it to.

Mindfulness meditation helps you manage your thoughts

without succumbing to the associated emotions. It empowers you to teach your mind to think differently so that your behavior is not negatively impacted. With continuous practice of mindfulness meditation, you will discern the true nature of thought empowering you to manage, control, and transform them for your advantage rather than your disadvantage.

Developing Focus & Discipline

Mindfulness meditation helps you develop focus and discipline. The reality is that all of us are capable of focus and discipline because the modern-day life calls for these elements willingly or unwillingly.

We have to get to work on time. We have to get to the station on time to catch the train. We have to reach the airport on time to ensure we don't miss the flight for an important meeting. We have to get the kids to reach school on time. And, many, many more instances of contemporary modern life make us stay focused and disciplined whether we like it or not.

With mindfulness meditation, focus and discipline can almost become second nature to you, and then, there will be no situation where you will not like to be focused and disciplined. So, how does mindfulness meditation sharpen your focus and discipline?

For every meditation session, you rely on your discipline to sit at the allocated place in the allocated time to prepare yourself for the session. You use focus and discipline to remain as still as possible as you focus on your breath or any other chosen anchor.

Each time your mind wanders, you employ the powers of your focus to bring it back to the present moment. Each time a judgment forms in your mind about a particular thought, you use your focus and discipline to ignore it, and compel yourself to remain a witness to the thought.

Mindfulness meditation helps to clear the clutter from your mind freeing it of wasteful thoughts so that your power to focus on productive work improves. Mindfulness meditation requires tremendous focus and discipline to practice consistently, and as you keep practicing, these elements become more powerful just as the strength of your muscles increases as you keep exercising.

Self-Awareness

Self-awareness is the ability to delve deep within yourself to connect with your true self. It goes beyond knowing your likes and dislikes, understanding what kind of skin you have or what kind of personality you have.

Self-awareness is knowing our core emotional, spiritual, and physical self. Why is self-awareness so important? Because it helps us understand what our body, mind, and spirit truly want to live a completely fulfilling and meaningful life. Self-awareness is also a complete acceptance of who and how we are without judgment. It helps us understand how and why we behave in a particular way in any given situation and also gives us insights into how we can change ourselves for the better.

Meditation is the perfect solution to increase self-awareness. As you focus on your thoughts, emotions, and feelings, and peel them layer by layer, you will be able to see yourself for what you truly are – with absolute zero judgment.

For example, suppose you are at a loud party, and you appear to be enjoying yourself with dance, drink, and food. The external atmosphere could be driving you to enjoy the party. Move away from the noise, people, and the electrifying atmosphere of the party, and ask yourself, "Are you really happy in this place?" The answer you get in the silence without the effects of the external atmosphere and from the depths of your heart will be as close to the truth as possible.

Mindfulness meditation in a quiet and peaceful place will help you truly understand what your heart and mind want. Being happy or sad is easy for everyone. Knowing exactly what gave you happiness or sadness requires self-awareness. As your self-awareness increases, you can navigate our behaviors and actions more towards what is good for you and less towards what is not.

During mindfulness meditation, you learn to observe and track your strengths and weaknesses in an objective way which increases your self-awareness significantly. Other benefits of self-awareness include:

Being at peace with ourselves – When you observe and accept yourselves for what you truly are, you are at peace with yourselves. You clearly understand the reasons for your sadness, happiness, and other emotions, and find ways to align your body and mind to the situation.

Improved clarity in communication - As your self-awareness increases and you understand yourself better, you will able to articulate your thoughts in a much better way than otherwise. Your own clarity is passed on via the power of communication and speech.

Improved decision-making capabilities – Knowing your true self will help you make the right kind of choices that are aligned with your core values and principles. You will find it easy to quickly decide whether something or someone is suitable for you or not.

Clarity of your life purpose – When you become self-aware, you know the exact direction you need to take to achieve your life purpose. Increased self-awareness clears up the pathway and shows you exactly where you want to be and what you want to achieve.

Mindfulness meditation is a fabulous way to improve self-awareness and take advantage of all the benefits of knowing yourself truly well.

In this chapter, you learned crucial personality traits that you will develop through the continued practice of mindfulness meditation. You learned about how mindfulness meditation helps you:

•   To live in the moment for an enriching, immersive, and fulfilling life

•   To become non-judgmental so that you can learn from all kinds of experiences in your life

•	To understanding and interpret the true nature of your thoughts so that you can transform them for your benefit

•	To develop focus & discipline resulting in increased efficiency and productivity

•	To be self-aware so that you can follow your dreams and life purposes in a way that suits you best.

Chapter 9. How to Increase Focus with Mindfulness Meditation

Let's start by trying to understand what focus actually is. Focus can be generally defined as the act of paying attention to what is necessary (important) while avoiding what is unnecessary (unimportant). In this chapter, we will look at focus in the context of our day-to-day mental activities (more commonly known as "work"). We will get a glance of what it feels like to have complete focus, how it can improve our lives, some of the common reasons people lose focus and finally, how mindfulness can help improve our focus levels.

What a focused mind feels like

Have you ever seen a laser in real life? A proper laser can emit light so focused that it can cut through solid steel! On the other hand, a bulb also emits light but can hardly burn anything, much less cut through steel. This is the difference between a focused mind and a distracted mind.

A focused mind has the ability to process information, filter out unnecessary options and get to the goal in the fastest route possible. It is very similar to the phenomenon of "flow" or "tunnel vision" or "being in the zone".

Benefits of Having Focus

I don't think you need to be sold on the importance of having focus. If you are already convinced about this, I suggest you skip to the next section. However, if you're curious about what practical benefits focus can bring to your life, here are a few you can get by building a ninja-like focus.

Benefit #1: You will get things done faster. Obviously, we're referring to the mental tasks and activities that you need to finish with your brain. Improving focus might not increase your deadlift capacity. But if you put in the time and effort to develop focus, you will slowly start noticing something strange. Other people tend to take much longer time to finish the same tasks than you. Also, what seems easy to you will appear like a mammoth task to them.

Benefit #2: You will get better at problem solving. Human progress is measured by the scale of problems we are able to solve. The ancient man was able to solve the problem of food and staying warm. In the modern age, we have solved the problem of gravity i.e., going to the moon and beyond. All of this happened because we honed our problem-solving skills. With increased focus, you will be able to objectively define the problem, identify the issue and filter out irrelevant fixes to end up at the right solution. This process involves a lot of critical analysis and paying attention to what is required and ignoring what's not. Notice how this is precisely what focus is about, according to our stated definition.

Benefit #3: You will feel more positive. Getting more work done and possessing the ability to control your attention will make you happier. Nobody likes being distracted. Even more so when we know that we're supposed to be working on our tasks. By developing focus, not only can you finish your tasks faster, but you will also feel better for being able to evade and avoid distractions like a pro. This creates a positive feedback loop where you feel good for staying focused which develops your ability to stay focused which in turn makes you feel even better.

Why we lose focus

Attention is a depleting mental resource. There can be a lot of reasons for losing focus depending on your psychology and circumstances. Listed below are 2 of the most common reasons for losing focus in our day-to-day life.

Reason #1: Distractions

Studies have shown that will power and focus are actually finite resources. This means that the more distracted you are, the tougher it is to get your focus back. This is especially true in the current age of internet and social media. This goes to show that being exposed to distractions and social media in particular can be detrimental to our brain's performance when it comes to cognitively demanding tasks.

In his book Deep Work, author Cal Newport writes that the ability to focus on hard tasks is becoming increasingly rare and valuable at the same time. This means that the people who can figure out how to develop and maintain focus amidst the distractions will thrive in our economy.

Reason #2: Lack of energy

We have all experienced this. You can rarely focus on work when you're exhausted physically and/or mentally. Your brain needs high levels of oxygen and fuel to get the energy it needs to function properly. Although you can develop and maintain focus while being unhealthy, the best results are obtained when your body is physically fit. They don't say "A sound mind in a sound body" for nothing. A healthy body will produce the right levels of hormones to balance the stress of mental wear out. From personal experience, I can say that being physically fit by doing regular exercise has given me a natural boost in productivity and my ability to focus. In the book The Power of Full Engagement, authors Jim and Tony point out that the key to peak performance (both physical and mental) is energy management. High achievers balance energy expenditure with intermittent energy renewal through optimal relaxation. It pays to learn how to invest your energy well.

So, if you are able to spike your energy levels and avoid distractions, you will find that the intensity and duration of your focus increase rapidly.

How exactly Mindfulness can build your Focus

We have already understood that being distracted is one of the biggest reasons for losing focus. If you can eliminate distractions to your brain, you have effectively won half the battle. Here is how mindfulness can help you avoid and deal with distractions.

Think of your attention as a muscle. The more you train

it, the better it gets. When you're being mindful, you practice living in the present moment. That means you're training your brain's neural network to prioritize paying attention to the current moment over the past or future(distractions). By repeatedly bringing your attention back to the present moment, you get good at avoiding distractions. The more mindful you are, the more focused you are on the present moment. This is in line with the definition of focus which is paying attention to the important and avoiding the unimportant.

Once you get good at mindfulness, you can translate that developed focus into any field. This is because you are still paying attention to the present moment but just different forms of it. Instead of paying attention to your breath, you will be paying attention to the object of work like a book or a presentation or a software.

A paper published in Psychiatry Research Neuroimaging Journal has shown that practicing mindfulness meditation leads to increase in the brain's gray matter density. For the unaware, gray matter is the part of the brain that handles various functions such as sensory perception, self-control, decision making etc. People with denser gray matter can learn better, memorize faster and most importantly, maintain focus on important tasks for much longer duration.

Bonus tips to increase Focus

Bonus Tip #1: Chew gum. Seriously. As mentioned on a podcast by Scientific American, chewing gum increases oxygen flow to your brain and also injects some insulin into your blood resulting in higher focus.

Bonus Tip #2: Find a line of work that is both interesting and important to you. This has to be genuinely passionate for you and demand your undivided attention. Otherwise, your brain activates a default network that switches your attention to other stimuli.

Bonus Tip #3: No more multi-tasking. One task at a time, fellas. In reality, our brain cannot pay attention to more than one thing at a time. So, people who think they are multi-tasking are actually switching their attention between different tasks rapidly. This has been shown to fray your brain out and reduce productivity levels.

Bonus Tip #4: Observe your body's natural energy rhythm and align your work accordingly. Your brain is usually very active just after breakfast and at dusk. So, schedule your heavy-lifting tasks during those times and maybe take a power-nap or go for a walk during the afternoon. Also, don't forget to take breaks in between work sessions, get ample sleep, eat nutritious food and exercise regularly for best results.

Chapter 10. Meditations for Everyday Life

Your brain is always rehearsing something. The more you say, "I hate my body" or "I'm dumb," the better your brain gets at believing that. The more you get angry in traffic or judge other people who look or sound different, the stronger that neural pathway gets. Your mind is like your social media feed. You get to decide what to block and what to follow. Whatever you follow will affect you (consciously or unconsciously) and influence how you see yourself and the world. Mindfulness lets you see and decide which habits you want to build and which you want to eliminate.

Finding Your Passion

One of the greatest joys in life is finding your own passion. It also happens to be a huge stressor, because you don't always know what you want to do, and you get a million messages about what you should or shouldn't do. Meditation can help you find some clarity about what you really love. It can also help with creativity, because you can let go of fixed ways of thinking and explore the world as it appears in that moment.

1.Find a comfortable posture and take a few deep breaths. Notice how it feels to breathe and be in your body.

2.Let your breathing be natural and focus on how you feel. Use your breath or sound as your anchor and rest your attention there.

3.When you're ready, let go of the anchor and allow your attention to be with whatever is predominant in your awareness.

4.If whatever you're noticing lasts for only a moment or two, just notice it and then let it go. But if it sticks around, try to pay attention to it as you would your breath, sound, or body sensations. See if you can be interested and curious about this experience just as it is. Notice it with all of your senses. What can you see, hear, smell, taste, and touch? What happens as you explore this stimulus?

5.When that sensation or stimulus disappears, come back to your anchor until another prominent experience arises for you to explore.

6.Once you've practiced this for a bit, you might gently

ask yourself, "What do I really love to do? How does x or y make me feel? Is this something I want to work at no matter what anyone else says?" You don't have to try to answer these questions—let them be there and notice what happens as you bring them to mind. You can let them percolate for hours, days, or even weeks. See what arises when you don't need to force an answer.

7. As you finish, take a few more deep breaths and notice how you feel now.

AM I DOING THIS RIGHT?

Both finding your passion and meditation require a degree of letting go and trusting yourself. You don't have to know everything or have all the answers. It doesn't have to make sense. And it won't always feel all that nice. The idea is that you'll want to work at it because it makes a difference overall.

The Everyday Stuff Practice

You almost certainly have stuff in your life you'd rather not deal with. Doing chores, helping out with siblings, or working late—necessary tasks you'd prefer not to do. The key is to just do the activity, notice what your body feels like as you do it, and see if you can find something to be curious about, without adding resistance or commentary to it.

1.Wherever you are, take a moment to pause and recognize; then recognize and let go of any stories, judgments, or critiques.

2.Take a few deep breaths and let your body settle as much as possible.

3.Letting your breath be natural, place your attention in your body, particularly in your feet. Notice what it feels like to stand, even bending your knees a bit to feel more grounded.

4.As you engage in this everyday task at hand, try to keep your attention in your body, finding something to hold your interest. It might be how the steering wheel feels beneath your fingers or how the lawn mower vibrates in your hands while you cut the grass.

5.Your mind will likely keep wanting to make a story out of this task ("Why do I have to do this? No one else is working this hard."). Try to let those thoughts come and go, then come back to the feeling of your body in this place.

6.If you start to get annoyed or frustrated with the

people around you, you might try sending them some kind thoughts (here). Send yourself some, too, if you feel particularly stuck in negative thinking.

7.As you finish, take a few deep breaths and notice what it feels like to be free of your usual frustrations with this activity.

TAKE IT FURTHER

If you start doing this practice regularly, you'll notice the same stories or judgments come up a lot. So when you're standing in line somewhere, instead of getting caught up in the whole "Why is this taking so long? I always pick the wrong line" story, you can just notice that thought as a thought, and then come back to this present moment where all you are really doing is standing, feeling your feet on the ground, and breathing. This frees you from the unhelpful habits you didn't even know you were building.

Seeing Past Differences

No one sees the world the same way you do. Everyone gets their unique perspectives from their own beliefs, backgrounds, experiences, values, parents, education, and more, which is pretty incredible when you think about it. Your perspective is completely unique to you. And while most people do their best to be nonjudgmental about others, it can be hard to identify with people who have different backgrounds, look unfamiliar, or have different values.

This practice helps you recognize your own perspective. It helps you see some of the judgments you might not even know you're making about other people and lets you focus on the things that you have in common with people who seem different, rather than the things that divide you.

1.Find a posture that feels comfortable and take a few deep breaths, feeling the breath go in and out of your body.

2.Let the breath be natural.

3.Check out how your body and mind feel right now.

4.When you're ready, bring someone to mind who feels different from you. That might be based on how they look, act, or sound; a group they belong to at school; or simply what you think of them.

5.Try to let go of your thoughts about this person or interactions you've had. Instead, simply picture this person and consider what you both have in common as people. What makes you both human? Just like you, this person gets scared and lost, feels wonderful, doubts herself, wants to be happy, etc.

6.Say to yourself:

This person has feelings, thoughts, a body, and a mind . . . just like me.

This person is doing their best . . . just like me.

This person makes mistakes . . . just like me.

This person wants to be happy . . . just like me.

You can make up your own words or phrases that feel right for you. Focus on what you share with this person. What makes you both vulnerable human beings trying your best?

7.Notice if this person feels more real after making these connections. Perhaps instead of being "a bad guy," you now see someone who is a fallible human, just like you.

8.Explore how this feels in your mind and body as you take a few more deep breaths.

TAKE IT FURTHER

You can pair this practice with the next one to help you deal with difficult or challenging people in your life—for instance, that kid in your class or person at work who drives you wild. Or when your siblings or parents just don't get it. It helps you recognize some of your automatic judgments or reactions about others, so you can have more say in how you relate to people who are both similar to and different from you.

Dealing with Difficult People

Whether it's at school, at work, on the bus, or in your own household, there will always be difficult people: people who don't like how you look, how you talk, or what you're doing—regardless of anything you do or who you are. Maybe this is because they're unhappy. Maybe it's because it's a full moon. The truth is, it's about them, not about you. As RuPaul says, "What other people think of me is none of my business."

We want to protect ourselves from difficult people, yet it helps to see that they're also struggling, just like us. This creates compassion and connection.

1.Pause. Breathe. Notice how it feels to be in your body.

2.Explore all of your senses in this moment without

needing to change or solve anything.

3.When you're ready, bring someone to mind who is a difficult person in your life right now, noticing what happens in your mind and body. Try to be gentle and compassionate with whatever occurs.

4.Pairing this practice with the previous one, Seeing Past Differences, notice what it's like to see this person as just another human being. Just like you, they feel lost, want love, and get confused.

5.Take a moment to recognize that, no matter what they are doing, it isn't about you. Even say aloud, "What they think of me is none of my business." That doesn't excuse pain they cause you, but it lets you get perspective. Their (wrong or hurtful) view of you doesn't diminish who you are.

6.Remind yourself that you can't control their actions, only your own response. You can notice what hurt feels like and then decide what you let affect you. (Feeling the hurt gently isn't the same as reacting to it or feeding it with angry thoughts.)

7.As you do this, come back to your body sensations and breath. Let those be your focus.

8.As you finish, take a few more breaths and notice how you feel.

9.When you're done, take a moment to either write down or consider aloud these questions: What do I need to do to care for myself? How does being with this person truly make me feel? Am I letting them dictate my emotions by reacting? What could I do when they start to really get to me?

BUDDY UP

At times, the healthiest thing is to protect yourself. A friend or family member can help with this. Talk to someone you trust in order to come up with a plan. Maybe you need to set boundaries or avoid the troublesome person. Maybe you choose to pause and feel your feet when a person you can't avoid gets to you. Sharing this with someone else helps you be compassionate with yourself and know you aren't alone.

Receiving Feedback

Getting feedback is a necessary part of your life. You get grades and test results at school, and evaluations at work, not to mention likes on social media. Yet it's likely no one has ever told you how to actually do this well.

You're just supposed to be okay with whatever people tell you. Often, that's not easy at all.

The idea here is to take what's useful, discard what's not, and respond rather than react. A compliment becomes a gift. You can receive it and enjoy it without needing to keep getting more or basing who you are on what other people think of you. And a critique is an opportunity to use what's helpful and then reject any part that makes it a personal comment on who you are.

1.Take a few deep breaths. If you've received a compliment or critique, this helps you pause, break with your automatic reaction, and choose a different response.

2.Let your breathing be natural. Feel your feet on the ground and the temperature of your skin.

3.If you've received a compliment, notice how it feels in your body. Experience what it's like to have something positive happen. Let yourself receive this compliment. If some part of you thinks you didn't deserve it, try to see that as only a thought and focus on—and feel—the good in your body with your senses. Soak it in as much as possible. You deserve it.

4.If you've received a critique, again pause and feel your feet on the ground. Concentrate on what's happening in your body, rather than any reaction in your mind. If it feels uncomfortable, can you notice how that discomfort feels without automatically reacting?

5.As you focus on your body, remind yourself that this isn't personal. It's not about you. Take in what's helpful in the feedback and then come back to your body. Ask yourself, "What can I learn from this? Can any of this help me once I've calmed down a bit?"

6.Explore any judgments about yourself or the other person as just thoughts coming and going.

7.If someone criticizes you personally, acknowledge that it isn't a helpful critique, but a verbal slap. Feel that discomfort in your body without reacting to it. Explore the Dealing with Difficult People practice to find a balanced response.

TAKE IT FURTHER

Sometimes, your brain needs to vent or share how it's reacting. There's a lot of momentum that comes up when you feel wronged. You don't have to ignore it. You can go for a run or write an angry letter, but don't send it—at least not until a day when you've cooled down to see if that's how you really want to respond.

Know Your Brain: Positive Neuroplasticity

With all the talk of stress and difficult emotions, it can seem like mindfulness focuses only on the negative. In fact, it's just as powerful to practice with the good stuff. Remember, the more your brain does a task, the stronger and more efficient the neural pathway for that task becomes. Whenever you notice contentedness, calm, peacefulness, delight, happiness, safety, comfort, or satisfaction, your brain gets better at recognizing them and making them a permanent fixture in your life.

Take time to focus on what you're good at, what you're capable of, and what you dream of doing. The more attention you pay to those moments, the more you'll notice them in the future. Every time you laugh with a friend, hear a good song, or eat something delicious, notice and savor those moments. Instead of focusing on how things could be different or what other people have that you don't, be mindful of what is working (you passed a test, assisted a goal, or helped a friend) and how you really are doing your best. Practice enjoying your achievements, even tiny ones like finishing a chapter in a book. You get to be in charge of growing your brain the way you want. Rather than thinking about meditation like medicine you take when you're sick, think of it like food that feeds your mind rather than your body.

Conclusion

Parents who take the time to teach their children mindfulness will notice benefits in their child's life, as well as their own. It teaches the ability to regulate emotions and form healthy social relationships. It can give them the self-esteem that they need to fight against mental bullies and the ability to understand their experience as it happens.

With all these things, your child will develop skills that can carry them through their entire lifetime. You might not be able to curb temper tantrums or emotional outbursts completely, but you will notice positive changes in your child.

Remember that mindfulness should be practiced regularly so that your child sees the most benefits from it. Only by practicing with you will your child have the instincts and skills to apply these exercises in difficult moments by themselves. Simply look forward to the wonderful development benefits that your child will see as they grow up. I hope your child enjoys these mindfulness exercises as much as my little girl. I do them with her all the time, and if I start to get too busy in my day, she reminds me!

Mindfulness is a great tool – all you have to do is use it. So what are you waiting for? Compile the exercises you want to use with your child and get to it! Mindfulness may not be able to solve all your problems, but it will sure put a dent in them!

Daily meditation practice can make you healthier, happier, and more successful than ever. Only a few minutes of meditation practice daily can help you lower stress, improve your mental and physical health, boost your focus and increase work productivity.

If you heard about meditation but don't know how to begin – or you have practiced meditation in the past, but need help to get started again, this beginner's meditation guidebook is for you.

Whether this is your first experience with meditation practice, or you have practiced before, this book will transform your relationship with yourself and the world around you. This book opens the door to a life lived in the freedom of your innermost being. We hope that this book is going to help you to find best method for mindfulness meditation, useful exercises and practices, good music suggestions for relaxation, stress relief and better sleep. We encourage you to try implementing meditation to your everyday life because we live in stressful time and our mental and physical health could depend on it.

www.ingramcontent.com/pod-product-compliance
Lightning Source LLC
Chambersburg PA
CBHW070702250726
48662CB00001B/224